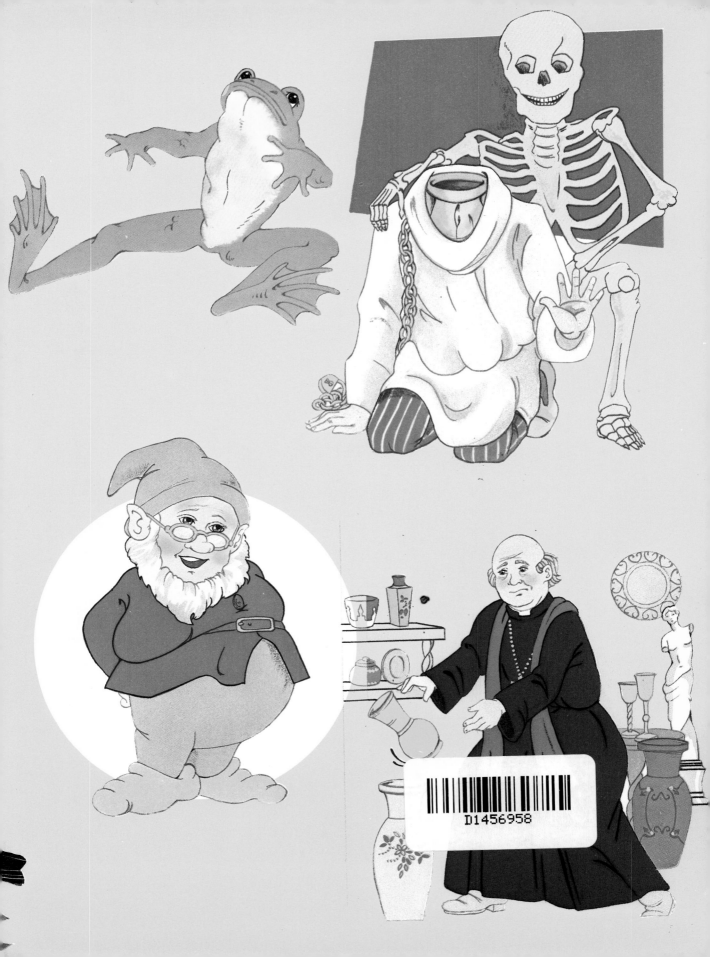

Contents

Published 1985 by Derrydale Books,
Distributed by Crown Publishers, Inc.

Five~Minute
Bedtime Stories

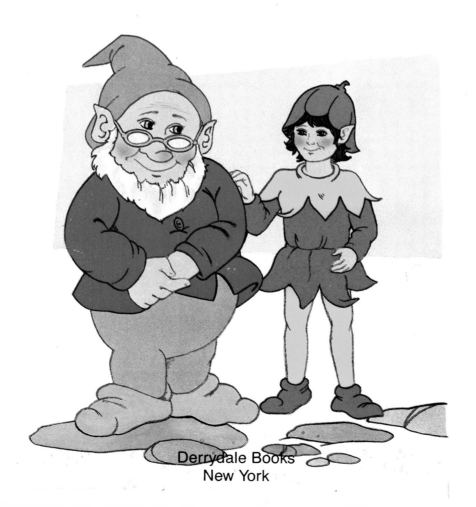

Derrydale Books
New York

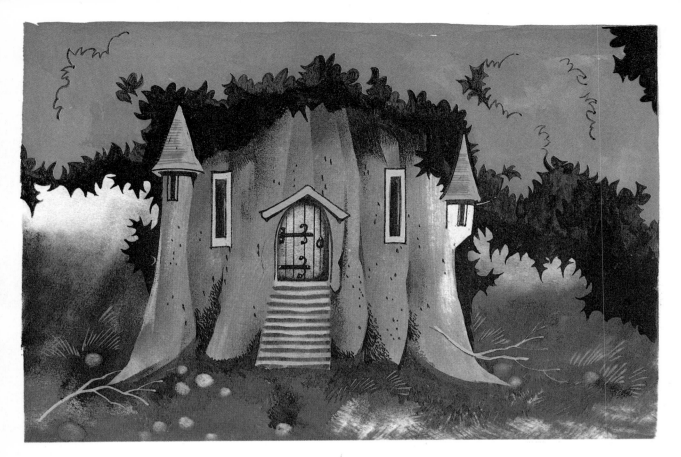

The Holly Bush Knights

by Ruth Hoult

The field mice were holding a meeting in the garden of Number 1 Chestnut Lane. It was the first garden where the country began.

They were sitting, standing, whisking tails, grooming whiskers, grooming fur, and squeaking one to another, while grouped around a forgotten story book, which lay open on the grass.

The picture was of a large castle. Men in armour stood on the battlements firing arrows and cannon balls on their enemies below.

The fieldmice had many enemies, among them Mr Cat O, Black the Weasel, Sly the Red Fox and Mr Barn the Owl.

"That is what we want," said Barley Mouse, "a castle. Then we would be safe from all our enemies."

"What a good idea," they all said. "Where shall we build one?"

"Shall we build our castle in the long, grey roots of the beech tree in Half Acre Field?" suggested Corn Mouse softly. "What a splendid fortress it would make."

But Barley Mouse didn't agree. "It is far too low," he said. "A castle should be high."

Rye Mouse had an idea. "The tall chestnut tree on Dragon's Hill," he said.

Barley Mouse shook his head. "High enough, yes," he said. "But there are no holes in the trunk to make a shelter. We can't live among the branches. What will happen when the cold times come, and all the leaves fall, and little white bits come out of the sky and cover the ground? What will we do then?"

Wheat Mouse stepped forward very importantly.

"We all know what we need," he said. "And the very thing is right under our nose. It's high and the leaves don't fall in the cold time. The holly bush in this garden."

"Yes, the holly bush," they all agreed.

The holly bush had light green leaves tinged with gold like sunlight at the edges. Its branches came right down to the ground, and all around it grew a bank of purple heather.

It was the very place . . . for what could be better than prickly holly leaves for keeping enemies away?

"We will call it Holly Bush Castle," said Barley Mouse. "And we will be the Holly Bush Knights."

The soft, brown earth floor, under the holly bush, was the armoury.

Wheat Mouse was busy making suits of armour out of walnut shells.

Rye Mouse was making spiky helmets out of the hard, green cases of horse chestnuts.

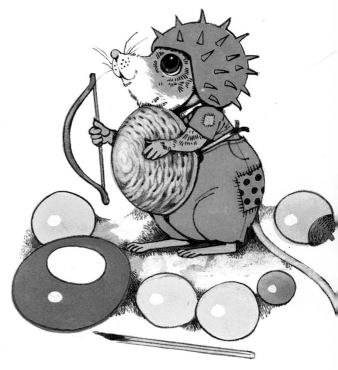

Corn Mouse was stocking up the horse chestnuts themselves for cannon balls; also acorns, and cherry stones, and stones. In fact, anything that was hard, and small enough to go inside the cannon.

Barley Mouse was making the cannon. He had a cardboard tube mounted on a tin lid. A piece of bamboo cane rammed down the barrel was the firing pin.

"It is all very scientific," Barley Mouse said.

Beet, Kale and Mustard Mouse were making arrows from matchsticks and lollipop sticks. And bows from small branches fallen from the silver birch tree.

They had found some green garden twine to make the strings.

In their storerooms the lady mice kept a feast of food, stored in old yogurt cartons which someone had thrown away.

Soon the news of Holly Bush Castle began to spread far and wide. For it is impossible to keep a secret in the bird and

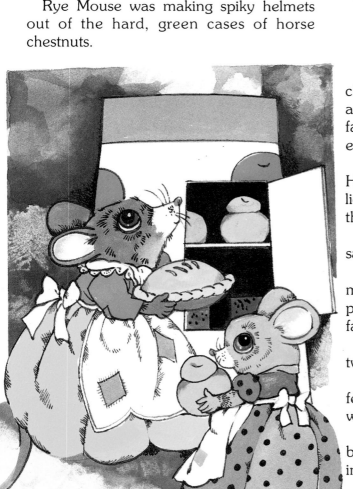

animal world. There are too many sharp eyes and ears about.

"Have you heard," sang Speckle the Thrush, *"of the Holly Bush Knights."*

Mr Cat O, who was preening his whiskers, pricked up his ears.

"They live in the holly bush, Number 1, Chestnut Lane," sang on Speckle the Thrush.

"Oh, do they?" said Mr Cat O to himself. "I must pay them a visit. It is a long time since I had a nice juicy mouse for my supper."

The Holly Bush Knights watched Mr Cat O approach. Mr Cat O thought he was being very clever as he sneaked round the holly bush to find a place where he could hide in the heather.

"I will be ready to spring on the first mouse who comes out," he said, licking his lips greedily.

Inside the holly bush, Beet Mouse was giving orders.

"Take aim, mice," he said. "Fire."

A shower of matchsticks and lollipop sticks came hurtling through the leaves and landed on Mr Cat O. *Thud, thud, thud, thud.*

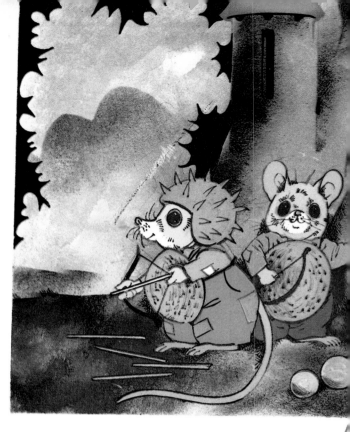

Mr Cat O stood up and shook himself angrily.

"Take aim, mice. Fire," ordered Beet Mouse again.

Another shower of matchsticks and lollipop sticks came hurtling between the leaves to fall on Mr Cat O.

Mr Cat O had had enough. He shook a paw at the holly bush and slunk away defeated.

"Have you heard of the Holly Bush Knights," sang Speckle the Thrush. *"They defeated Mr Cat O."*

Black the Weasel listened.

"They live in a holly bush, Number 1, Chestnut Lane," finished Speckle the Thrush.

"Oh, do they?" said Black the Weasel to himself. "Thank you, Mr Thrush, for telling me. I must pay them a visit. I can't remember when I last had a nice little mouse for my supper."

Black the Weasel appeared at Holly Bush Castle.

"Hello," he called. "Anyone at home? It's a lovely evening for a chat."

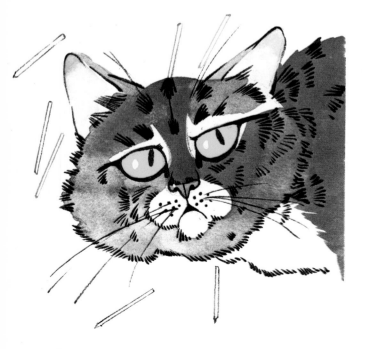

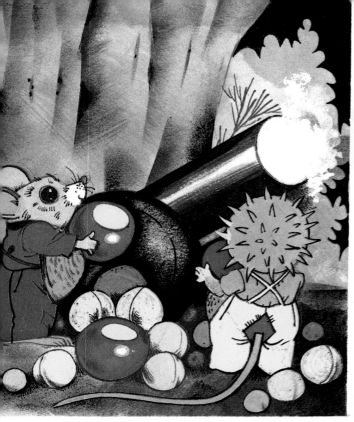

A shower of matchsticks and lollipop sticks came from between the leaves and stuck into Sly the Red Fox's fur.

He brushed them off with his paw.

"You can't hurt me with your sticks and your stones," he told them. "I am going to sit here and wait, even if it takes a day, for you to come out to look for food. Then I will catch you."

"It is going to be a siege," said the lady mice of the castle.

"Oh good," said their children. "We can eat the feast in the store rooms."

Sly the Red Fox sat outside and sat outside. In the end he had to give up. The Holly Bush Knights had won.

"Have you heard of the Holly Bush Knights," sang Speckle the Thrush.

"They defeated Mr Cat O, Black the Weasel and Sly the Red Fox."

Mr Barn the Owl, sleeping in a nearby ivy-covered tower, woke and heard.

"Indeed," said Mr Barn the Owl. "Then I must see them. Where do they live?"

"They live in a holly bush, Number 1, Chestnut Lane," finished Speckle the Thrush.

"I will go tonight," said Mr Barn the Owl.

But the Holly Bush Knights were not deceived by these friendly words. They knew Black the Weasel; he was very cunning.

Barley Mouse had his mice ready before the cannon.

"Take aim, fire," he commanded.

Horse chestnuts, acorns, stones, cherry stones, came hurtling between the leaves onto Black the Weasel. And the largest horse chestnut hit his nose.

Black the Weasel turned and ran.

"Hurrah!" shouted the Knights of Holly Bush Castle.

"Have you heard of the Holly Bush Knights," sang Speckle the Thrush. *"They defeated Mr Cat O and Black the Weasel."*

Sly the Red Fox pricked up his ears.

"They live in a holly bush, Number 1, Chestnut Lane," sang on Speckle the Thrush.

"Oh, do they?" said Sly the Red Fox. "I think I might pay them a little visit. I just fancy a mouse or two for my supper."

Sly the Red Fox went to Holly Bush Castle and sat outside.

"Take aim, fire," ordered Beet Mouse.

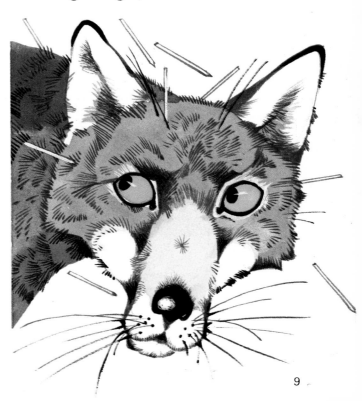

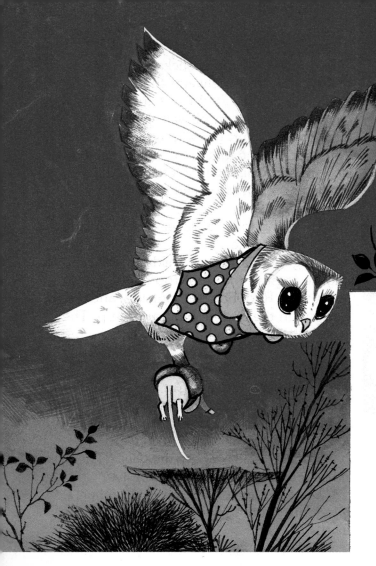

"It will be nice to have a fat juicy mouse for my supper."

When it was dusk Mr Barn the Owl flew silently over the fields to the garden of number 1, Chestnut Lane, and came to rest on the branches of a silver birch tree. And waited.

The Knights of Holly Bush Castle did not know he was there. And one by one they came out in search of food to replace their stores after the siege by Sly the Red Fox.

Mr Barn the Owl winged silently down and snatched up Wheat Mouse in his claws.

He flew back to the silver birch tree and lowered his bright yellow beak at Wheat Mouse. But Wheat was wearing his walnut armour. And Mr Barn the Owl couldn't break it.

Mr Barn the Owl dropped Wheat Mouse to the ground with disgust. He flew away in search of something easier to eat.

All the other mice gathered round Wheat Mouse.

"Are you all right?" they asked

"I am fine," replied Wheat Mouse. "My armour saved me from Mr Barn the Owl and it helped to break my fall, too."

"Hurrah, hurrah," chanted the Knights of Holly Bush Castle.

"Have you heard of the Holly Bush Knights," sang Speckle the Thrush.

"They defeated Mr Cat O, Black the Weasel, Sly the Red Fox and now Mr Barn the Owl."

And this time there was no one to take up the challenge of the Holly Bush Knights. They had won their last battle.

"They are famous," finished Speckle the Thrush.

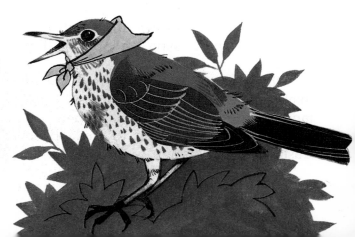

The Birthday Present

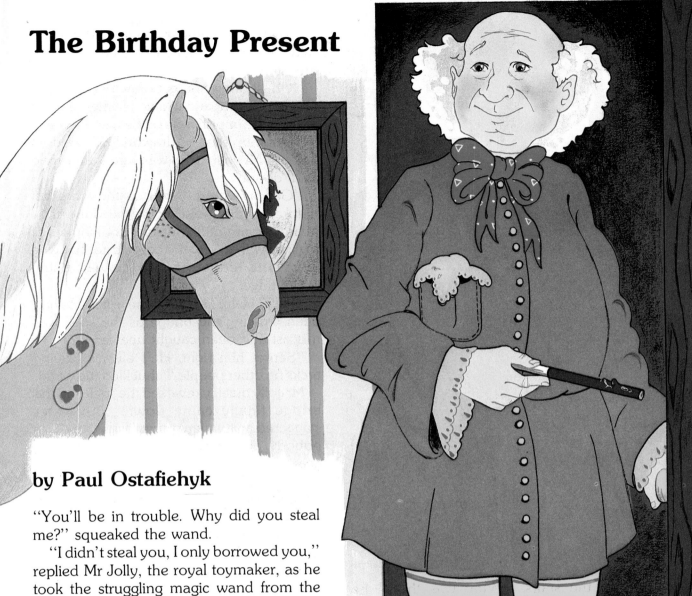

by Paul Ostafiehyk

"You'll be in trouble. Why did you steal me?" squeaked the wand.

"I didn't steal you, I only borrowed you," replied Mr Jolly, the royal toymaker, as he took the struggling magic wand from the inside pocket of his brightly-coloured jacket.

"You should wait for the high sorcerer to return from lunch before you do anything," warned the wand.

"The king commanded me to make a rocking horse for the prince's birthday and to keep it a secret. It's in the room at the top of these stairs, and I'm going to use you to cast a spell to make sure nobody can get near it," panted Mr Jolly as he climbed the steps of the palace's north tower.

Ignoring the protests that were still coming from the wand, Mr Jolly stood confidently outside the room. He poked his chubby face around the door to make absolutely certain that the splendid present was still there. When he saw that it was, he closed the door and waved the magic wand through the air. "Seal the door and let no one see the secret," commanded the toymaker.

Mr Jolly expected some sort of flash of light or a bang. He covered his head with his arms to protect himself, but when nothing happened he crept forward and gently touched the door. ZAP! A strange tingle shot through his hand. With a cry of alarm he leapt backwards and almost tumbled

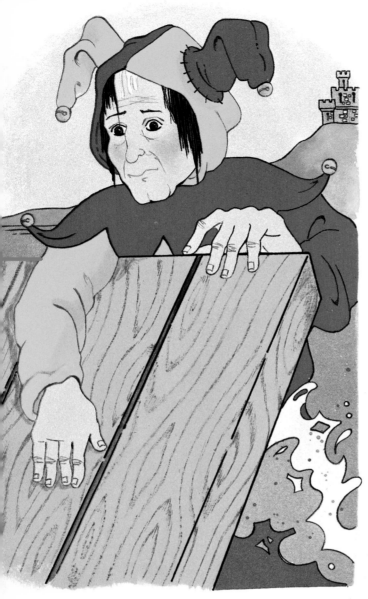

"There's something you should know," said the wand as Mr Jolly waved it through the air.

"Oh, shut up and get on with it, wand," ordered the impatient king. Neither of them noticed the impish tone of the wand's voice.

"Open up the . . . drawbridge?" said an amazed Mr Jolly, who was sure that he had said 'door'.

"Get on with it," snorted the king, but before anything else could be done they heard a commotion outside. Looking out of a window they saw the court jester hanging from the edge of the slowly rising drawbridge.

"Help! Help!" shouted the jester. He had been crossing the bridge as the spell was miscast and been caught unawares.

"Serves him right. He's always playing tricks on other people," chuckled the wand.

Mr Jolly quickly reversed the spell and the bridge finally came down. The jester staggered away, very puzzled, as there was nobody anywhere near the bridge lifting gear.

"Ha, ha! I tried to tell you, but you wouldn't listen," tittered the wand. The king scowled at Mr Jolly.

"The first spell that you cast made you say the wrong word. The spell is foolproof," explained the wand.

down the stairs. "What was that?" he gasped.

"Electricity," replied the wand, although the question had not been directed at him.

Mr Jolly did not know what electricity was, but his puzzled look soon gave way to a smile. "Most satisfactory. I knew I could do it. I've seen the sorcerer do it many times. It was almost too easy," boasted a pleased toymaker.

Just then the king bounced up the stairs. "Come on then, let's have a test ride," he said to Mr Jolly, who only just stopped him touching the door.

"Just wait while I reverse my locking spell," he said.

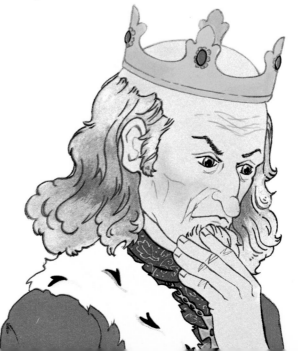

Not to be beaten, the king sent the toymaker for the magical battering ram. Although it had not been used for a very long time its magic was renewed every year by the high sorcerer. No gate could withstand just one knock from the golden ram's head.

As Mr Jolly struggled up the stairs with the ram he wondered what would happen if they could not reach the horse. The last time the king was angry the toymaker was forbidden to eat any pudding after dinner for a month. This month's pudding was strawberries and cream, which he liked best of all.

"On the count of three we'll ram the door," said the king, helping Mr Jolly with the ram.

"One, two, three . . . charge!" he yelled at the top of his voice. As they ran towards the door Mr Jolly closed his eyes. BOI-OING! The ram's head had turned into a great spring just before it hit the door. The king and the toymaker were sent tumbling backwards down the stairs.

"Oh, I wish the king was riding the horse!" said Mr Jolly, shaking the wand angrily.

Quick as a flash the king was sitting on the horse at the top of the stairs.

"How did that happen?" asked Mr Jolly.

The wand was about to answer, but the high sorcerer had appeared from nowhere and was standing by the horse. He cast a spell to take away the wand's voice as a punishment for its mischief.

"The spell kept everything out of the room, but didn't stop things coming from the room, as you found out," smiled the sorcerer.

"When your majesty has finished the test ride I'll put the horse back. The room will be ready for 'ordinary' use in one or two years when the spell wears out. Then you might like to join me for tea, it's strawberries and cream," said the sorcerer, winking at the lucky Mr Jolly.

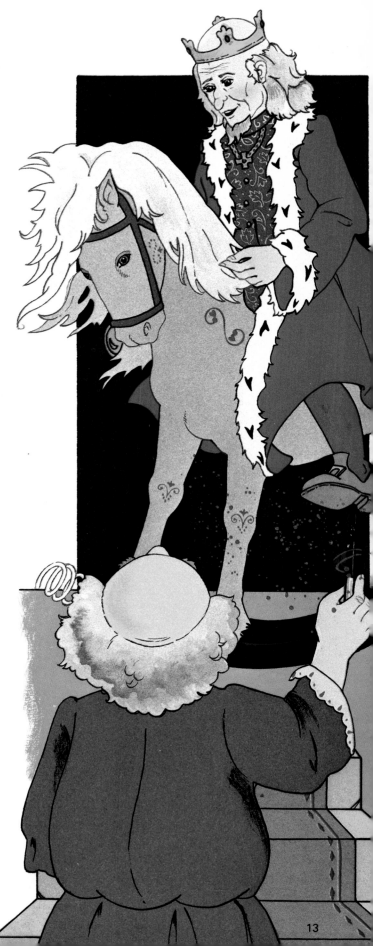

13

The Pigeon Candlestick

by G. Ford

One day a real live pigeon with shining purple and green feathers came to the windowledge to pick up some crumbs. The sun shone on the candlestick, and all at once Perry Pigeon saw the china pigeon at the top.

He dropped the crumbs and stared and stared. "What a lovely little china pigeon," he thought, and knew right away that she was the one he wanted to share his nest.

Every day he came to look in at the window. But it was no good, for she was made of china. He forgot to eat, he lost his bright colours, and his feathers drooped. His friend Willie Wizard was quite upset. "Whatever is the matter, Perry?" he cried.

On the mantelpiece of a big room in a big house stood a lovely china candlestick. It was shaped like a Christmas tree with china branches reaching right to the top.

Little china pigeons sat quietly on each branch and there was space for a candle between each bird.

When the candles were lit, the china birds seemed to come alive.

At the top fluttered one pigeon all alone, with wings outstretched. She was so pretty that people cried out, "Oh, what a lovely little pigeon!" whenever they saw her.

Perry pointed to the pretty bird inside. "All day she just looks out at nothing," he explained sadly. "Oh, if only she wasn't made of china."

"For goodness sake, don't worry about that," said Willie quickly. "You're always finding my magic stick for me when it gets lost, so now it's my turn to help you." And off he went to get his stick, the magic stick that did such wonderful things.

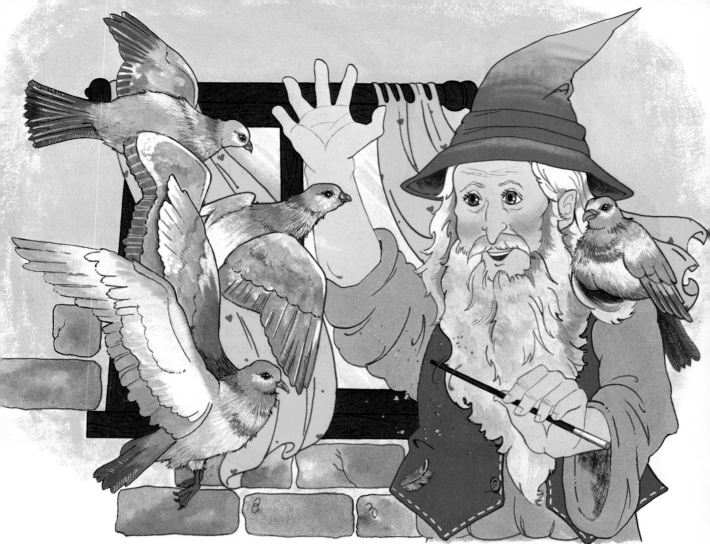

Willie often forgot things because he was always trying to help so many people. The last time the magic stick was lost, Perry had had to fly all over the British Isles to look for it, up hill and down dale. And then he found it behind Willie's own back door!

At last Willie returned. "I found it right away," he said with a chuckle. "It was behind the kitchen door again."

With the stick in his hand they were soon inside the big house. "Come to life! Come to life!" cried Willie, waving the wand. But he made one little mistake, for ALL the pigeons came to life, as well as the pretty one at the top, and there was such a flurry of wings and *coo-coo-coo* calls that you'd have thought a whole pigeon house was let loose.

"No, no," gasped Perry, who was nearly knocked over in the rush. "I don't want them all. Just the little pretty one." And he pushed and pushed through the excited birds, until he managed to get beside her, and drew her gently to his side.

Willie hurried to correct his mistake. "Back to your places, please," he said, waving the magic stick once more. They pushed and squeezed and fluttered back to their places, all except the little pigeon from the top of the pigeon tree.

Perry led the little one towards the window, and soon they were flying high above, towards the bright blue sky, winging their way towards happiness.

Willie Wizard watched them go with a happy smile. Then he blew some pigeon fluff from his waistcoat and hurried home to get his supper.

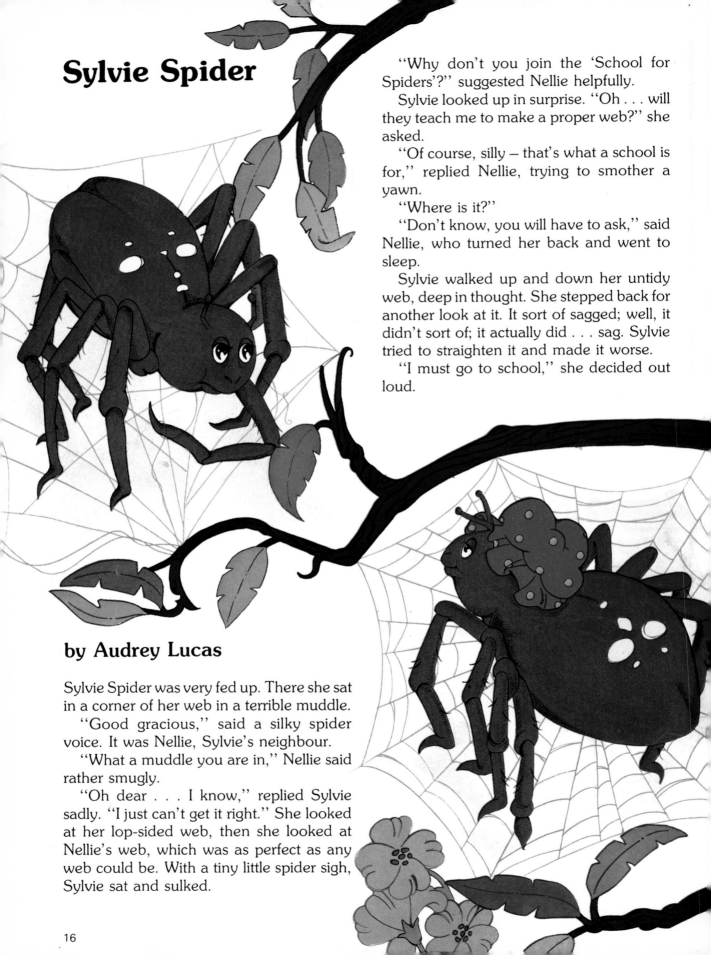

Sylvie Spider

"Why don't you join the 'School for Spiders'?" suggested Nellie helpfully.

Sylvie looked up in surprise. "Oh . . . will they teach me to make a proper web?" she asked.

"Of course, silly — that's what a school is for," replied Nellie, trying to smother a yawn.

"Where is it?"

"Don't know, you will have to ask," said Nellie, who turned her back and went to sleep.

Sylvie walked up and down her untidy web, deep in thought. She stepped back for another look at it. It sort of sagged; well, it didn't sort of; it actually did . . . sag. Sylvie tried to straighten it and made it worse.

"I must go to school," she decided out loud.

by Audrey Lucas

Sylvie Spider was very fed up. There she sat in a corner of her web in a terrible muddle.

"Good gracious," said a silky spider voice. It was Nellie, Sylvie's neighbour.

"What a muddle you are in," Nellie said rather smugly.

"Oh dear . . . I know," replied Sylvie sadly. "I just can't get it right." She looked at her lop-sided web, then she looked at Nellie's web, which was as perfect as any web could be. With a tiny little spider sigh, Sylvie sat and sulked.

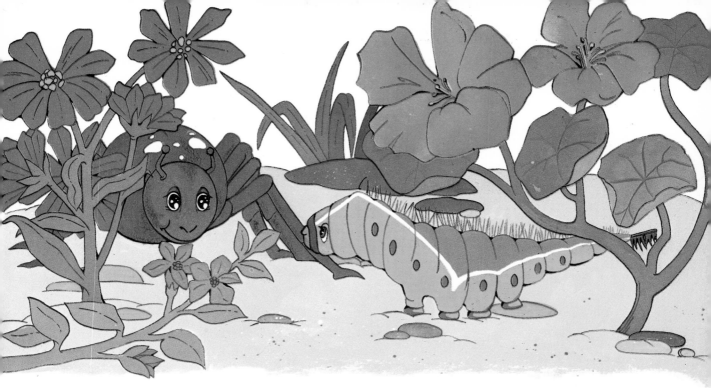

"Goodbye Nellie," Sylvie called to her neighbour.

"Goodbye, Sylvie . . . good luck," answered Nellie sleepily.

On the way to find the School for Spiders, Sylvie met a handsome caterpillar. He was bright green and gold with lots of fluffy feathers on his back. His name was Clarence.

"Good morning," said Sylvie to Clarence.

"Oh, good morning," he replied, "nice day."

"Yes, it is . . . em, could you please tell me where the School for Spiders might be found?" Sylvie asked.

Clarence thought for a moment. "Yes, I can, as a matter of fact," he said, looking rather puzzled. Sylvie quickly explained why she needed to go to school.

Clarence was very understanding. "I'll go with you if you like," he offered kindly, and the spider and the caterpillar set off straight away.

They stopped once, for lunch. Sylvie offered Clarence some of hers, but Clarence politely refused and munched happily on a leaf.

After the two friends had travelled some distance, they came across a beetle named Bertie. Bertie wore a shiny black overcoat. "Hello," he said, "where are you off to?"

"School," replied Sylvie and Clarence together.

"Mind if I come along?" asked Bertie.

"Not at all." So off they went. 'It's nice to have company when starting school for the first time,' thought Sylvie.

"Mia-ow, mia-ow!" Oh dear! The spider, the caterpillar and the beetle stopped in their tracks.

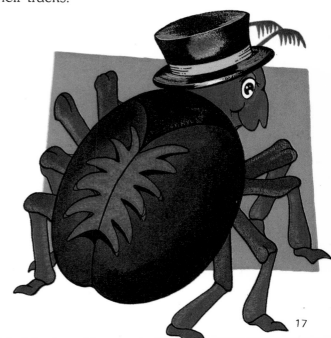

17

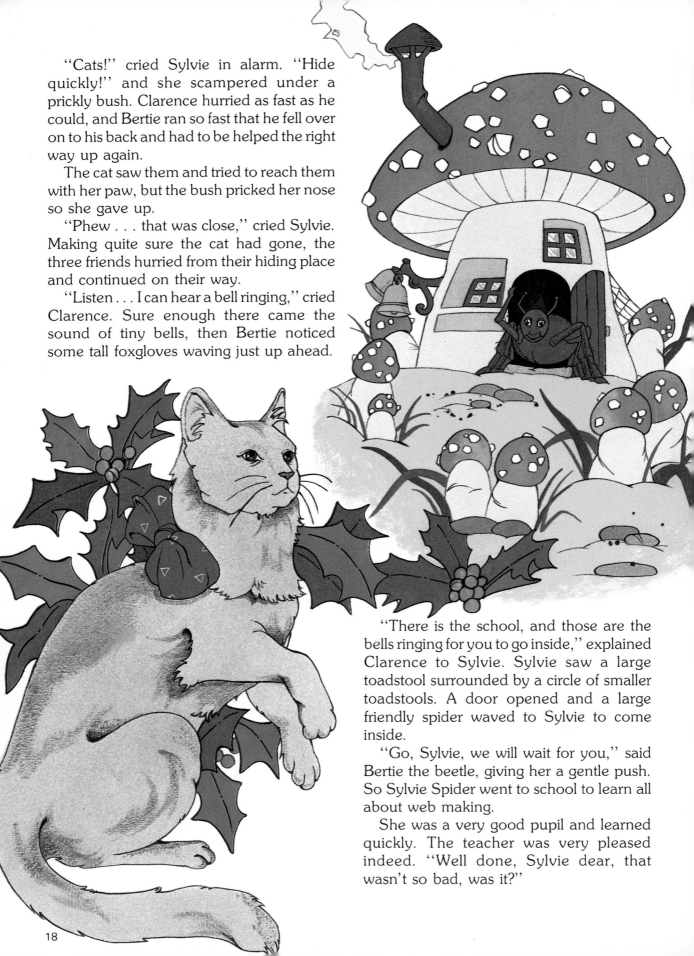

"Cats!" cried Sylvie in alarm. "Hide quickly!" and she scampered under a prickly bush. Clarence hurried as fast as he could, and Bertie ran so fast that he fell over on to his back and had to be helped the right way up again.

The cat saw them and tried to reach them with her paw, but the bush pricked her nose so she gave up.

"Phew . . . that was close," cried Sylvie. Making quite sure the cat had gone, the three friends hurried from their hiding place and continued on their way.

"Listen . . . I can hear a bell ringing," cried Clarence. Sure enough there came the sound of tiny bells, then Bertie noticed some tall foxgloves waving just up ahead.

"There is the school, and those are the bells ringing for you to go inside," explained Clarence to Sylvie. Sylvie saw a large toadstool surrounded by a circle of smaller toadstools. A door opened and a large friendly spider waved to Sylvie to come inside.

"Go, Sylvie, we will wait for you," said Bertie the beetle, giving her a gentle push. So Sylvie Spider went to school to learn all about web making.

She was a very good pupil and learned quickly. The teacher was very pleased indeed. "Well done, Sylvie dear, that wasn't so bad, was it?"

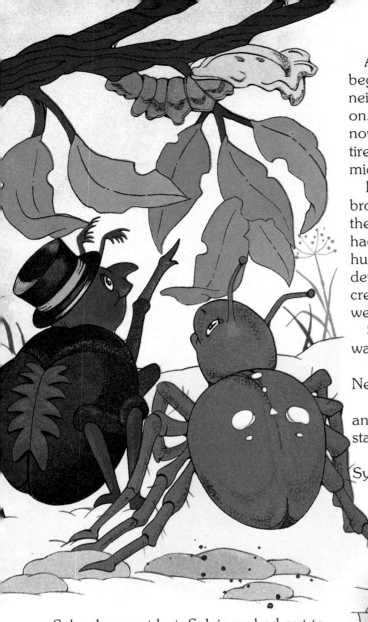

As soon as she arrived home Sylvie began to weave a new web. Nellie her neighbour was all agog to see how she got on. At last Sylvie's web was finished, but by now it was too dark to see and Sylvie was so tired that she fell fast asleep right bang in the middle.

It rained in the night, but morning brought the sunshine. It shone brightly on the young apple tree where Sylvie Spider had chosen to weave her web. There it hung among the apple blossom, covered in dew and sparkling like a jewel. All the little creatures of the gardens and hedgerows were gathered around to admire it.

Sylvie woke up from her slumbers and was so very proud of herself.

"Well done Sylvie," said her neighbour Nellie.

"Well done indeed," came a soft voice, and looking around Sylvie found herself staring at a beautiful butterfly.

"Why Clarence, is that really you?" cried Sylvie, her happiness truly complete.

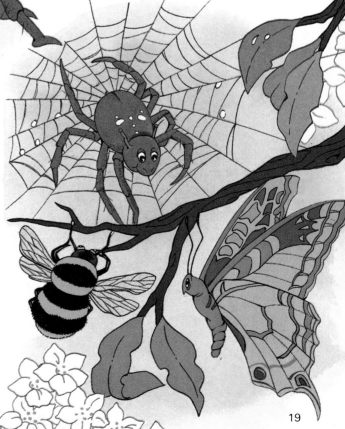

School over at last, Sylvie rushed out to find her friends. She could hardly wait to tell them how she had got on.

"Where is Clarence?" asked Sylvie, looking all round.

"Not here," replied Bertie, "he has gone to change." He pointed to a twig above his head. There was no sign of Clarence, instead there hung a rather sticky brown chrysalis.

"Oh no," cried Sylvie sadly, "I shall miss him so."

"Don't be sad," said Bertie kindly, "soon he will turn into a beautiful butterfly, and he will not forget you."

Jamie and the Exiled Dragon

by Paul Ostafiehyk

Jamie the farmer's son was walking home from school one afternoon when he saw something falling out of the sky. *Splash!* It plunged into a nearby pond and soaked him.

When he had stopped coughing and spluttering he saw a small green dragon sitting in the now half-empty pond. It didn't look frightening and was none the worse for its fall. Jamie wasn't even surprised when it spoke to him. "Hello, my name's George. What's yours?" inquired the dragon, his scaly eyes twinkling.

"Jamie. Where did you come from?" said Jamie.

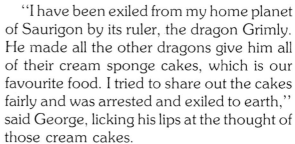

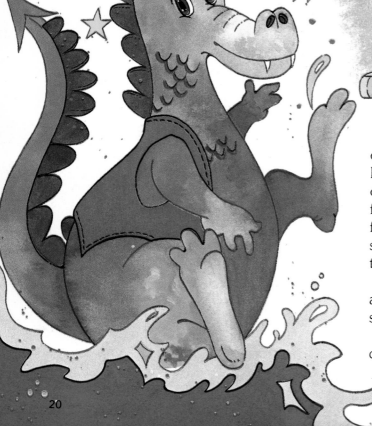

"I have been exiled from my home planet of Saurigon by its ruler, the dragon Grimly. He made all the other dragons give him all of their cream sponge cakes, which is our favourite food. I tried to share out the cakes fairly and was arrested and exiled to earth," said George, licking his lips at the thought of those cream cakes.

"Will you help me to return to Saurigon and free the other dragons?" asked George, still sitting in the pond.

"Yes of course," replied Jamie. "What do you want me to do?"

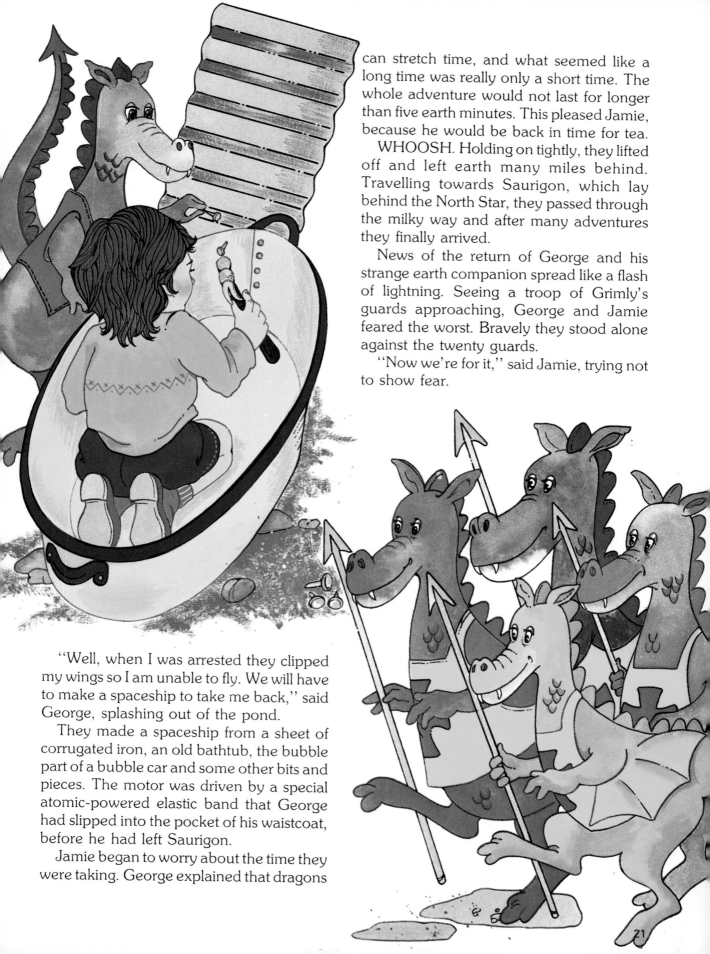

can stretch time, and what seemed like a long time was really only a short time. The whole adventure would not last for longer than five earth minutes. This pleased Jamie, because he would be back in time for tea.

WHOOSH. Holding on tightly, they lifted off and left earth many miles behind. Travelling towards Saurigon, which lay behind the North Star, they passed through the milky way and after many adventures they finally arrived.

News of the return of George and his strange earth companion spread like a flash of lightning. Seeing a troop of Grimly's guards approaching, George and Jamie feared the worst. Bravely they stood alone against the twenty guards.

"Now we're for it," said Jamie, trying not to show fear.

"Well, when I was arrested they clipped my wings so I am unable to fly. We will have to make a spaceship to take me back," said George, splashing out of the pond.

They made a spaceship from a sheet of corrugated iron, an old bathtub, the bubble part of a bubble car and some other bits and pieces. The motor was driven by a special atomic-powered elastic band that George had slipped into the pocket of his waistcoat, before he had left Saurigon.

Jamie began to worry about the time they were taking. George explained that dragons

21

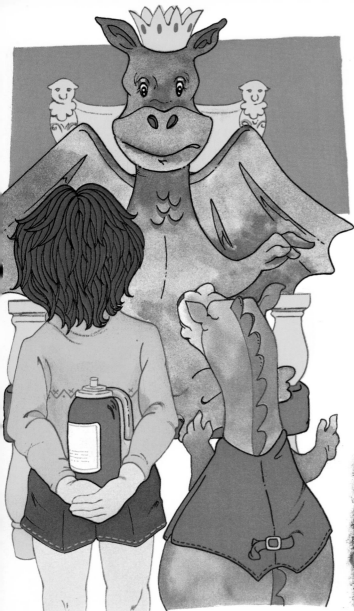

never again to be so greedy. He had given away his hoard of cakes and now spent most of his time baking them for others with his fiery breath.

After he had been introduced to Jamie, who was trying to hide the fire extinguisher he had brought along 'just in case', Grimly gave a party for the two heroes. He gave George a new set of wings. They all had a splendid time and when it was over George flew Jamie home. George said that he would visit Jamie soon and then flew back home.

Back in his own home Jamie couldn't make his mother believe what had happened. If she *had* believed him she would have known why he hardly touched his tea. On the way back he had eaten one of Grimly's delicious cream sponge cakes and was quite full. . . .

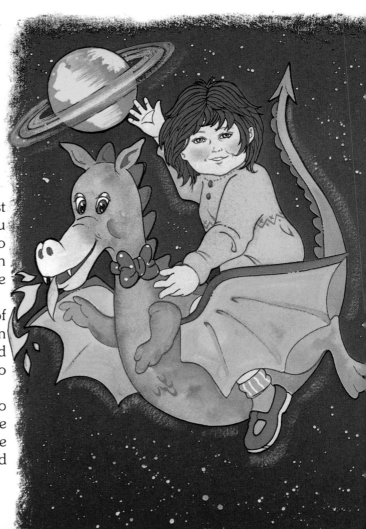

"Welcome home George, we were just organising a rescue party for you when you arrived back. The king would like you to come with us so that he can ask your pardon for exiling you," said the captain of the guard.

"How do I know that it's not some sort of trick?" asked a wary George. But when some of the crowd that had gathered reassured them that all was in order, the two adventurers were escorted to the palace.

Grimly had been very ill from eating too many cakes. He had turned a ghastly purple so that he looked like a large, over-ripe plum. When he at last recovered he vowed

The King's Clock

by Sheena Ronsey

"Oh, do stop whistling, Merriday," said the king crossly. "There's nothing to be happy about, and the Prime Minister is coming at ten o'clock to tell me the bad news."

"What bad news?" asked the Royal Wizard cheerfully. "How do you know it's bad news before you hear it?"

"It always is bad," snorted the king. "What's the time? I can't see the clock since my spectacles flew away."

Merriday looked at the clock and told the king it was a quarter to ten. It was a pity his spell on the spectacles had been a bit too strong.

"Why did you give them wings?" grumbled the king. "I only wanted them to jump on to my nose, so that I would not have to get out of bed to find them in the morning."

"I'm sure they'll fly home one day," said Merriday.

The wizard hummed a song about flying machines until the king told him to stop. Then the Prime Minister arrived, and started telling the king all the bad news. Merriday was not listening. He was thinking out a new spell for the clock. It was a tall grandfather clock and too heavy to fly, so wings would not do.

"What's the time?" said the king, and he got out of his chair to go and look at the clock.

The Prime Minister opened his mouth to

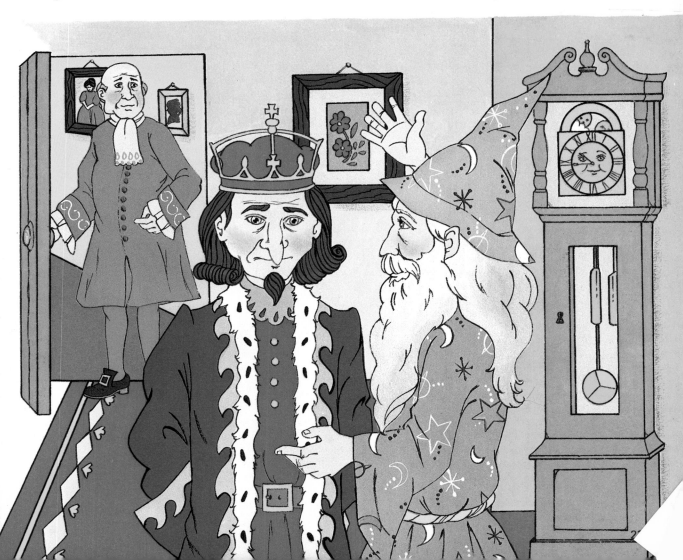

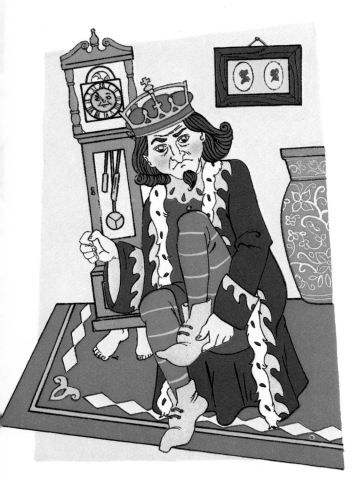

Merriday stopped smiling. He did not want to leave the palace and look for a job somewhere else. He was very sorry about the spectacles and the clock, and said so, but the king would not listen and the wizard had to go. He walked sadly out of the palace gate, but it was such a lovely day that he could not be sad for long. Very soon Merriday was singing a song about his grandfather clock, and thinking of all the places he would like to visit.

"How many miles to the seaside?" he asked a boy.

"Too many to walk," said the boy.

"Then I'll go by train," said the wizard, and he went into the railway station.

"You'll need another ticket for that clock," said the station master. "It's walking, so it must be a passenger, not luggage."

tell the king the time, but did not say anything, he was so surprised. Merriday had finished his spell. The clock stood up on two big flat feet and began to walk towards the king.

"Ouch!" yelled His Majesty when his nose suddenly met the wooden front of the clock, and, "Ouch!" again, when one of the big flat feet came down on his toe.

The Prime Minister frowned. The Royal Wizard smiled broadly because his spell had worked so nicely at just the right moment. The king hopped about on one foot, and he was very angry.

"Merriday!" shouted the king. "This is too much. First my spectacles fly away, and now my clock attacks me. You're sacked. I'll find somebody with more sense to be Royal Wizard from now on."

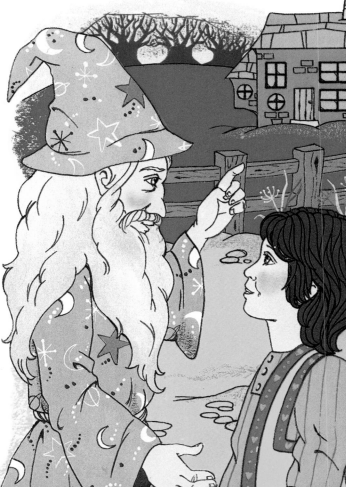

Merriday turned round in surprise, and there was the king's clock. It had followed him to the station and was trying to get past the ticket inspector without showing a ticket. The wizard told the clock to go home, but it took no notice of him. Then two policemen came running up and arrested the clock. One of them wanted to arrest the wizard for stealing it, but the other thought that was unfair, and while they argued about it, the train moved off with Merriday on board.

"I wonder why that clock followed me?" thought the wizard. "Perhaps it was sorry for making the king so cross with me."

Merriday enjoyed himself at the seaside, but when he got tired of being on holiday and looked for some work to do, he discovered that nobody wanted a full-time wizard. People were always pleased to see him, and they found little jobs for him, but nobody invited him to stay. He began to feel a bit sadder each day, as he went from town to town but could never go home, because he had no place to call home.

One day he was sitting in the sunshine half asleep when something landed on his nose.

"The king's spectacles!" cried Merriday joyfully. "Now I can go to the palace and take them back to the king. If I put the spell right, perhaps he will forgive me."

Merriday forgot that, since he was not Royal Wizard any more, he ought to go to the front door and ring the bell. He went in through the back door without even knocking, and hurried upstairs to the king.

"You are too early, Prime Minister," said the king. "I know you're early because the sun is not shining on my inkstand yet."

"Oh, I'm not the Prime Minister," said Merriday, "and I've got some good news to tell you. Here are your spectacles."

"That certainly is good news," said the king. He put on his spectacles and looked round the room to make sure they were still working properly. "Thank you, Merriday."

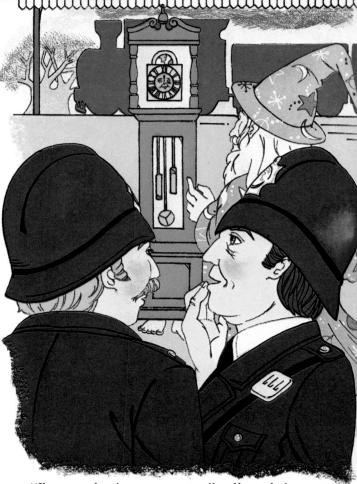

"I've made the wings smaller," said the wizard, "so they can't fly away again."

"I see it's raining," said the king, "so the sun won't tell me the time today."

Merriday looked at the king's clock, but it was saying half past three, and he knew that was wrong.

"The clock has stopped," said the king. "It tried so often to run after you that we had to tie it to the wall, and then it stopped. I think it's sulking because I sent you away."

The Prime Minister arrived and said he had some very bad news. "The new wizards have all failed their tests."

"Hooray!" shouted the king. "That's good news. Merriday can be Royal Wizard again."

Suddenly there was a whirring noise from the clock. It struck twenty-seven, and the hands whizzed round until they came to the right time. Merriday started singing, and for once the king did not tell him to stop.

Witch's Brew

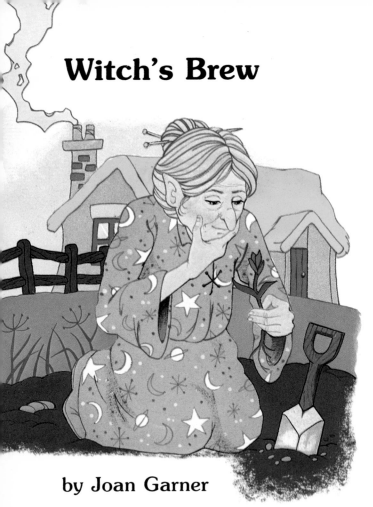

by Joan Garner

The witch of Whissington was accident prone. Nothing she did ever went smoothly and all her spells had peculiar results. For instance, when the children in the village had chicken pox, she tried to help. The spots vanished but the children finished up with large green blisters. Once, in June, the blackbirds were eating the strawberries. After her magic, it was not the blackbirds which had gone, but the crop of strawberries! Then she fell over her broomstick trying to get it airborne, and broke her leg.

The villagers regarded her as a joke and did not go to her any more. This made the witch very sad. She was a kind person and wanted to help people.

One summer day she was weeding her herb garden when an elderly gentleman leaned over her gate and said, "Are you the witch?"

"Yes. Can I help you?" she replied eagerly.

His name, he said, was John Brown, and he lived nearby. He wanted to marry a lady who lived in Whissington, but he was afraid that she would think him too old. He took out a photograph of a handsome young man in army uniform. "I looked like this when I was twenty," he said. "Could you make me look like that again?"

"Of course I can," chuckled the witch. "Come in and have a glass of elderberry wine while I get things ready."

Delighted that somebody wanted her help, she bustled round collecting all that she needed — her wand, the spell book, and the ingredients for the charm. Then she took out the black cauldron and started to mix, all the time chanting magic words and waving her wand. Soon a fragrant smoke,

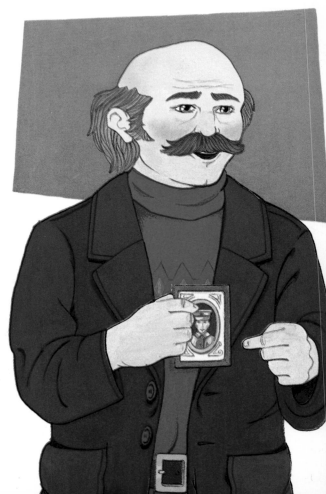

like a mixture of rose petals, honey and liquorice, rose from the cauldron. When the potion was ready, she handed it to Mr Brown. He drank it in one gulp and was transformed into a young man, exactly like the photograph.

Thanking the witch warmly, he rushed to the cottage where Miss Wright lived and asked her to marry him. Not surprisingly, she did not recognise him, but thought it was one of the village lads playing a joke on her. She pushed him out of the door, shouting, "I would not marry you if you were the last man on earth. I am going to marry Mr Brown, if he ever gets around to asking me."

So poor Mr Brown, having gone to all that trouble, found out that Miss Wright loved him as he was. He hurried back to the witch and asked her to reverse the spell.

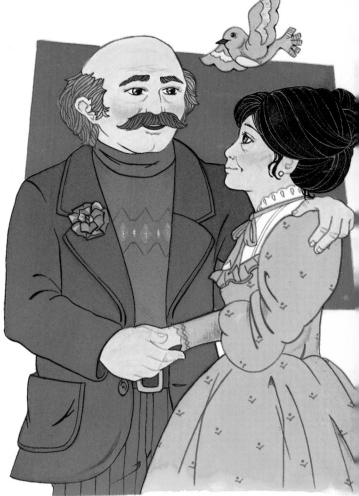

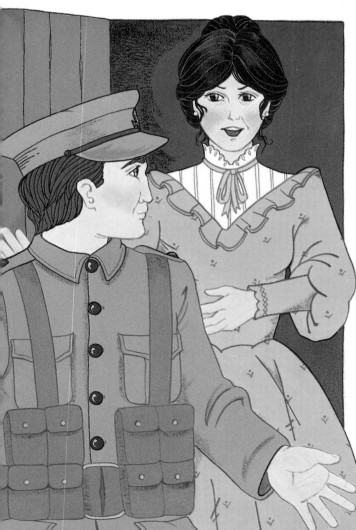

Sadly, she had destroyed the charm and was unable to chant the words backwards as was necessary. She did not dare risk anything other than the exact words, because there was no telling what age he would finish up.

Mr Brown went home, a sadder and wiser man. But, if you remember, nothing ever went entirely right with the spells, and this one only lasted twenty-four hours.

In the morning Mr Brown was back to normal. He hurried off to Miss Wright, proposed, and was accepted.

Mr Brown never confessed to his wife what he had done. But he did invite the witch to their wedding. She gave them her second best broomstick as a wedding present. It proved to be a very good sweeper, but had an unfortunate habit of flying out of the window on nights when there was a full moon.

Father Timoney's Problem

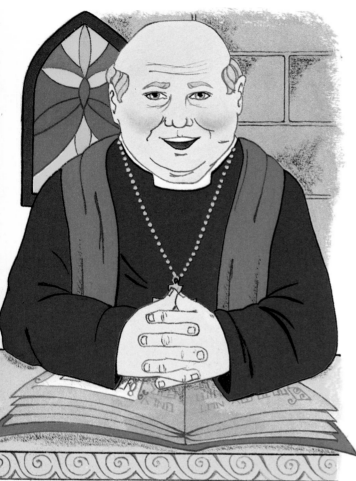

As he sat by his fire, a few days before the big party, he suddenly realised he had a problem. His fierce and extremely loud voice was sure to frighten the children.

He thought for a moment then stood up in front of the mirror. "Little children," he said, trying as hard as he knew to speak softly. But his words came out like a roar of thunder. He tried again and again.

"Oh dear," he thought, "I really don't want to scare the children. I love them so. But if I frighten them I'll never be asked back again."

Father Timoney made up his mind. He would ask all his friends how he could speak softly. Surely they could help. He started with old Doctor Jones.

by Jim Hewitson

Father Timoney, the parish priest of St Arthur's, had the loudest voice anyone in the town of Neston had ever heard.

His Sunday sermon shook the rafters of the old church and even people at the back of the church didn't doze long when Father Timoney began to speak.

And although he never told anyone, the priest was very proud of his loud voice, bawling out God's message.

One day, just before Christmas, he was asked to go along to the local children's home where he was to join in the carol singing and talk to the little ones.

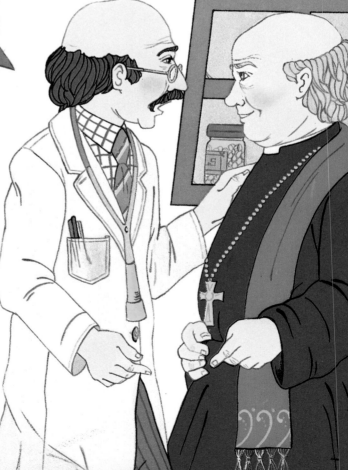

"Sorry, Father, this is a strange complaint. Sore throats, headaches and colds I can do," said the doctor. "But you have a loud voice and I don't think you'll ever lose it."

With a sigh Father Timoney left the surgery. Out in the street he saw Tom the coalman at the wheel of his lorry.

"Tom, how can I stop shouting?" asked the priest.

"Don't ask me, Father," said Tom. "It's the only way I know how to sell coal. A loud voice is no problem for me, in fact it's very important." And off he went bawling at the top of his voice: "Coal! Coal!"

Father Timoney turned into the zoo to speak to his friend Louis, the lion. When Father Timoney had a problem he often went to share it with his old friend — the king of beasts.

"I'd like to help," said Louis. "But

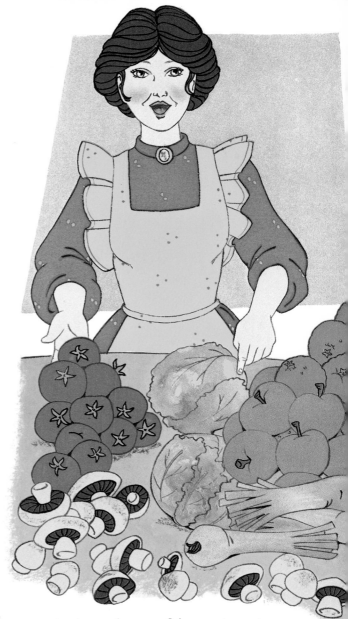

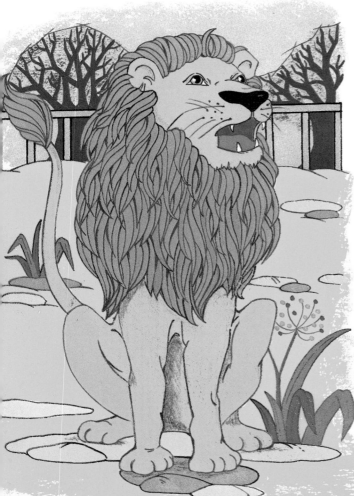

roaring is the only way I know to get my food. If I didn't roar that silly keeper would snooze all day in his shed."

Out in the town again the unhappy priest saw the vegetable stall with Mrs Leek busily shouting her trade: "Fresh fruit and vegetables! Lovely apples and oranges!"

Her advice was the same. "If I didn't shout I would never sell my wares, Father. I don't think I'm the right person to advise you."

Suddenly Father Timoney realised that his friends couldn't help. They needed their loud voices. He was in despair. He would have to cancel his visit to the children's

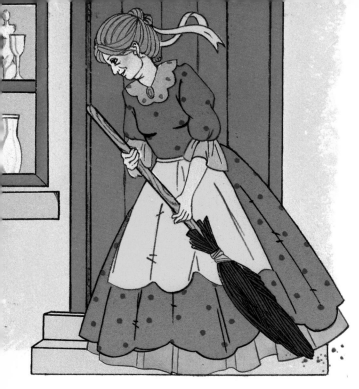

home. No one could teach him to speak softly.

Then, a few yards from the church in a narrow cobbled street, he passed the little shop which sold crystal vases, glasses and delicate ornaments.

Mrs Chandelier, the owner, was sweeping the doorstep. The priest nodded to her and when she asked why he was so sad, Father Timoney explained his problem.

"I think I might have the answer," she said, leading the priest inside. Row upon row of delicate vases and glasses lined the walls.

As soon as the priest's thundering voice rang out the glasses began to shiver on the shelves and Father Timoney had to leap and catch one as it tumbled floorwards.

"Come and spend a few afternoons in the shop. If you can't learn to talk quietly in here then you never will."

And so the priest went back three times. He sold glasses to the customers and between times raced around the shop to catch crystal sent spinning by his voice.

But slowly he learned to lower his voice and by the end of the week he was standing in front of the mirror in the chapel house.

"Little children," he began, and this time his voice was soft and gentle. The following day he joined the Christmas party and spoke so softly and kindly that the children asked him back the following week for tea and buns.

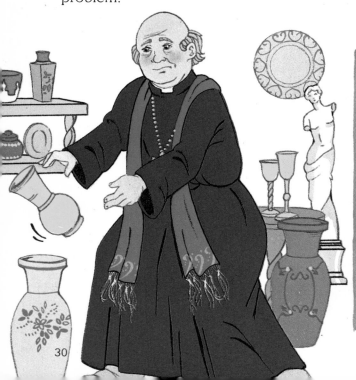

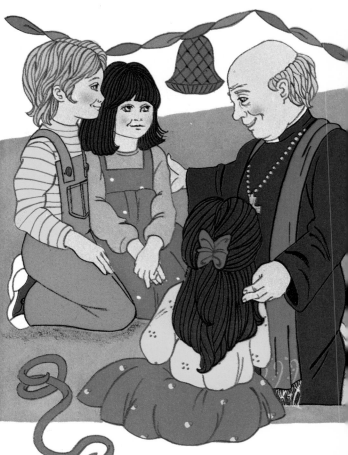

30

The Ghost Who Couldn't Haunt

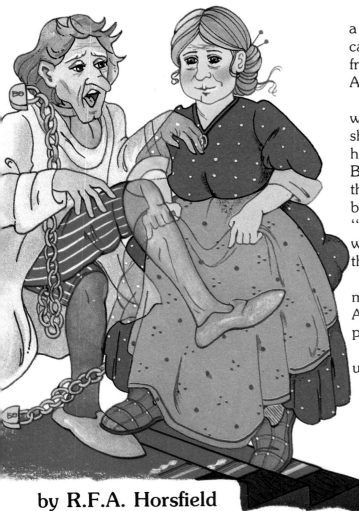

by R.F.A. Horsfield

With a bloodcurdling scream, Willy leapt out of the wall, right in front of the old lady who was making her way slowly upstairs. He waved his floppy white arms. He rattled his rusty chains. He uttered the most horrible moans and groans. He even took his head off and tucked it under his arm. But all to no avail. The old lady didn't even look at him. She just walked right through him and made her way along the landing. Willy tried again. He threw his head at her but, although his aim was good, the result was just the same. His head simply floated right through her and disappeared into the wall.

Willy groaned, this time in dismay. "What a rotten ghost I am," he said to himself. "I can't frighten anything. I couldn't even frighten a mouse, that's how rotten I am." And he started to look for his head.

He was on his knees, searching along the wall, when a bony hand fell suddenly on his shoulder and a gruesome chuckle echoed in his ears. Willy almost jumped out of his skin. But it was only Sammy Skeleton who stood there, rattling gently, a great big smile on his bony face. Willy breathed a sigh of relief. "You scared me stiff, Sammy," he said. "I wish you wouldn't creep up on people like that."

"Why, that's what I'm supposed to do, man," said Sammy. "I'm a ghost, aren't I? And what else do ghosts do but frighten people?"

"Well, I wish *I* could," replied Willy. "I'm useless. I can't even frighten the sauce off a

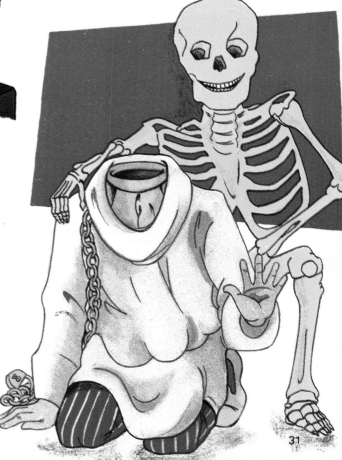

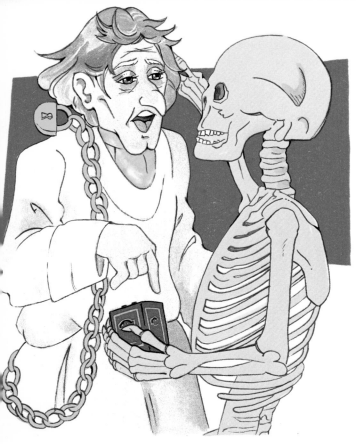

"Your battery, man. You knew you had a battery, didn't you?"

"Well . . . no . . . I . . . well . . ." muttered Willy.

Sammy Skeleton rolled his eyes. "Oh, man, where on earth did they find you?" He reached under Willy's white robe and came out with a little box. "Here it is! Now then, let's test it."

He placed his bony fingers on the terminals. "Just as I thought," he exclaimed, "nothing there at all. Flat as a pancake. Oh, really, Willy! You are the most stupid ghost! How on earth did you think you could give people a shock without a good battery inside you?"

Willy hung his head. But now, with his *new* battery, he is the most feared of all ghosts.

baked bean. And now I've even lost my head."

Sammy bent down and, passing his hand into the wall, he came up grasping the missing head which he placed on Willy's shoulders. "Well, there's your head, man. And do wipe that frightened look off your face. You know, the others are beginning to get a bit worried about you. You haven't given anyone a good scare since you've been here, and that's nearly a hundred years now. You're not earning your keep, Willy, and that's a fact."

Willy's shoulders drooped. "I know. I know. But I do everything right, don't I? I moan and I groan and I rattle my chains just like you told me to. The trouble is, they don't even see me. Or hear me. They don't even know I'm there."

Sammy shook his bones for a few minutes and thought it over. Then he said, "I've got it! I know what the trouble is. Here, let me have a look at your battery."

"M-my what?" stammered Willy.

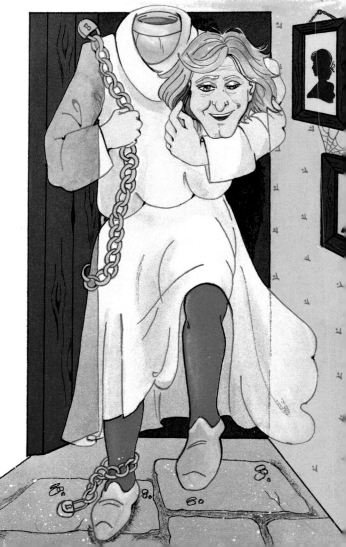

The Queen Who Could Not Clap

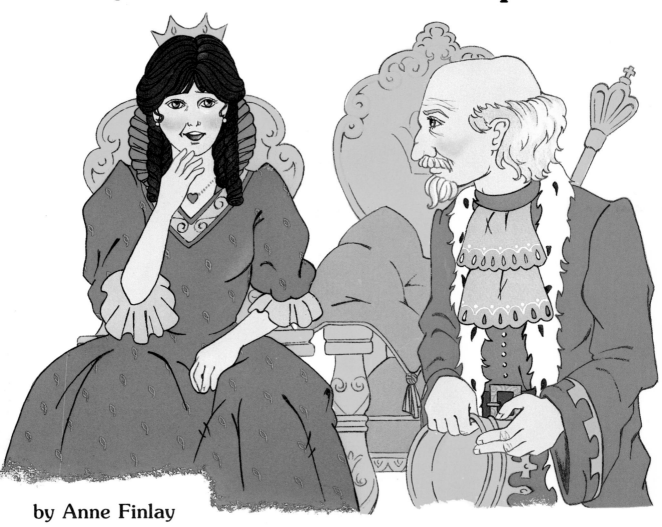

by Anne Finlay

"Ouch," said King Twig as his crown flew off his head and rolled down the steps of the throne.

He ran after the crown, caught it and put it back on his head.

"Really my dear," he said to Queen Blossom who was sitting on her throne beside him. "You will have to learn to clap properly or else sit with your hands on your lap at concerts. I can't have you knocking my crown off each time we sit on our thrones."

Queen Blossom had a problem. She could not clap. Each time she tried to clap her hands missed each other and did a lot of damage! She enjoyed concerts but if she sat in the audience no one sat beside her because once she had given a Duke a black eye when she had clapped very hard, and now the King didn't want her to clap when she sat next to him.

Tomorrow there was to be a very special concert and many important guests had been invited. Queen Blossom had a new pink dress with a long train to wear at the concert, and she was looking forward to it very much.

"Blossom," said the King kindly, "I must ask you not to clap at all, at the concert. I don't want anyone to be hurt."

"That will seem very rude," said the Queen.

"I am sorry, my dear," replied the King. "You must keep your hands on your lap and not clap at all."

Queen Blossom went out into the palace gardens. There the Royal Elves were picking bunches of flowers to decorate the palace for the concert. The Elves were busy, as usual, but they did notice that the Queen looked sad, and they wondered why.

When they had picked the flowers the Elves took them into the palace and asked one of the Footmen why the Queen looked so sad. The Footman told them about her problem.

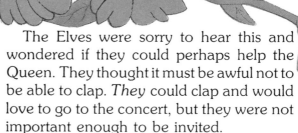

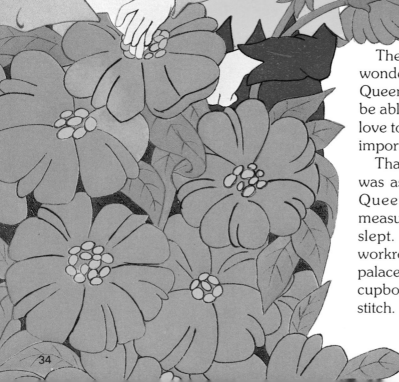

The Elves were sorry to hear this and wondered if they could perhaps help the Queen. They thought it must be awful not to be able to clap. *They* could clap and would love to go to the concert, but they were not important enough to be invited.

That night when everyone in the palace was asleep the Elves tiptoed down to the Queen's bedroom and very quietly measured the width of her hands while she slept. Then they hurried back to their workroom high up in the turrets of the palace. They got some pale pink silk from a cupboard and busily began to snip and stitch.

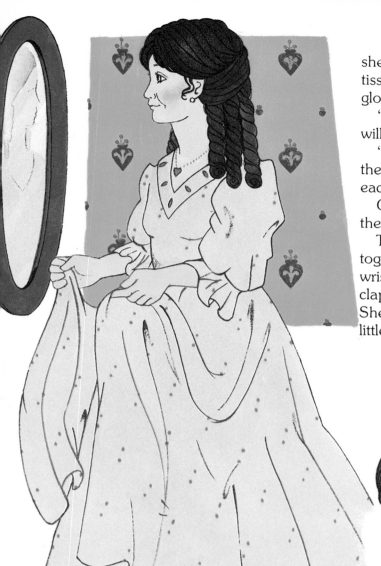

she opened it she saw lying in layers of tissue paper a pretty pair of long pink gloves, exactly the same colour as her dress.

"These are lovely," she said. "But how will they help me?"

"We have sewn a press-stud fastener to the gloves," said the Elves, "One part to each glove."

Queen Blossom tried on the gloves and they fitted perfectly.

Then she pressed the stud fasteners together and the two gloves joined at the wrists. Queen Blossom found she could clap quietly and politely like any other lady. She was overjoyed, and hugged the two little Elves, who blushed with pleasure.

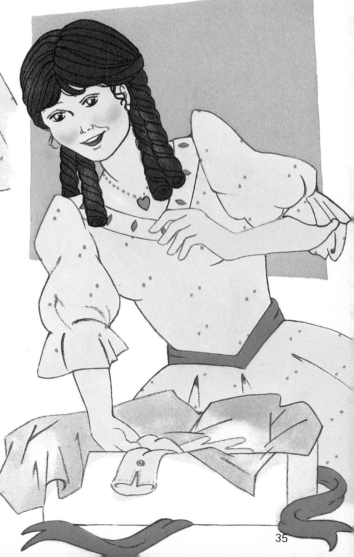

The next day the Queen put on her new dress to wear at the concert. She stood in front of the mirror and tried to decide which was the best way to carry the heavy train.

Just then there was a knock on her door. When she opened it there stood the Royal Elves carrying a long white box.

"Your Majesty," said the Elves, bowing low. "We heard about the problem you have when you want to clap and we have made something which we hope will help you."

"How kind and thoughtful," said the Queen. "Do come in."

The Elves handed her the box and when

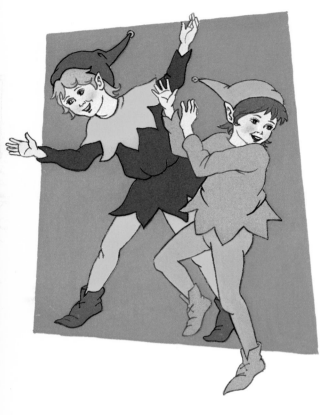

Then the Queen stood in front of the mirror and put on her crown. She swished the train of her dress back and forth while the Elves watched.

Then Queen Blossom turned to the Elves. "Would you like to go to the concert tonight?" she asked.

"Oh, Your Majesty," said the Elves. "We really would like to, but we are not important enough."

"Of course you are," said the Queen. "You shall be my trainbearers and help me with this long, heavy train."

The Elves jumped up and down with delight. "Oh, how lovely," they cried.

The concert was a great success. The Queen clapped happily and the King smiled proudly at his wife. Queen Blossom smiled at the two little Elves, who were having a wonderful time.

"Thank you," she whispered to them. "Now I shall always be able to clap."

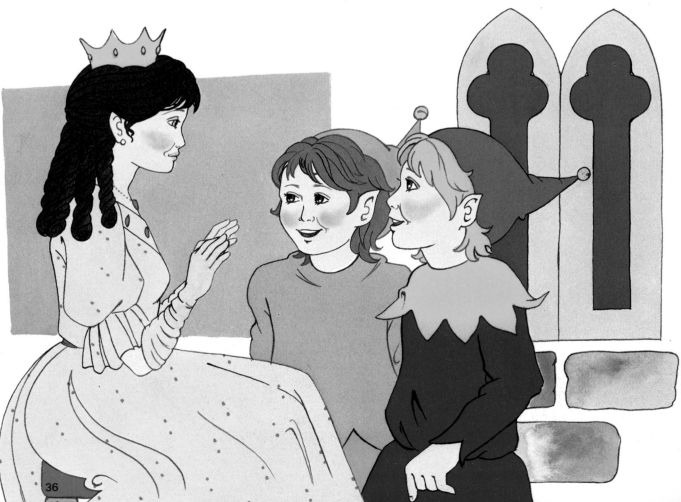

The Wizard and the Green Bubble

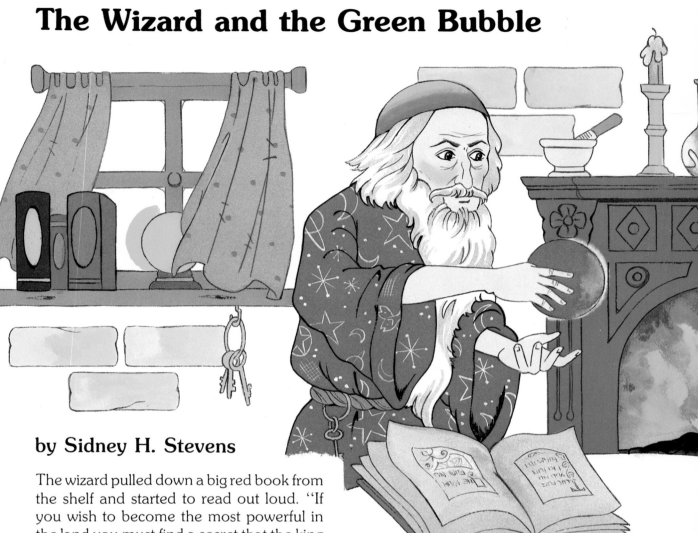

by Sidney H. Stevens

The wizard pulled down a big red book from the shelf and started to read out loud. "If you wish to become the most powerful in the land you must find a secret that the king cannot find. Should you fail, all your power will be lost and you will be turned to dust."

The wizard shut the book with a bang and began to mutter to himself. "Now, let me see, let me see — something that the king cannot find, but what?" He stopped suddenly and laughed out loud. "The green bubble! Of course, the green bubble, he can't possibly have one of those, can he?"

He called his messenger. "Take this message to the king at once," he said.

"Yes master," replied the messenger, and hurried off.

He soon reached the palace and asked for the king. "A message from the wizard, Your Majesty," he said, and held out the message.

The king took the message and started to read. "I have a green bubble," he read, "and now I am more powerful than you, for without a green bubble you have no magic." It was signed by the wizard.

The king laughed and tore up the message. "Tell your master," he said, turning to the messenger, "that I too have a green bubble, as you shall see."

He clapped his hands and a servant came. "Bring me the key to my store room," said the king.

"Yes, Your Majesty," said the servant, and off he went.

He was soon back with the key.

The king took the messenger by the hand. "Come, I will show you my wealth, and also the green bubble, then you can go back and tell your master, the wizard."

When they got to the store room the king unlocked the door. There, all laid out in rows, were hundreds and hundreds of bubbles of all shapes and sizes.

"My wealth," said the king. "Am I not indeed the most powerful in the land?"

The messenger was looking around. "But I can't see a green bubble," he said. "I don't believe you have one."

"Of course I have," laughed the king, "there must be one here somewhere."

But although they searched high and low not one green bubble could they find. There were white, black, brown, yellow, blue and red bubbles, but not one green one among them all.

The messenger laughed. "No green bubble, no magic," he said. "Go on, turn me into a frog."

The king tried, but it was no use.

"You see," said the messenger, "it's true!" And off he ran to tell his master.

The king was very angry.

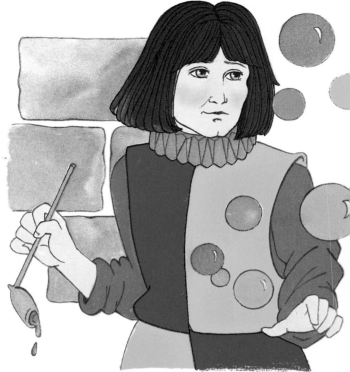

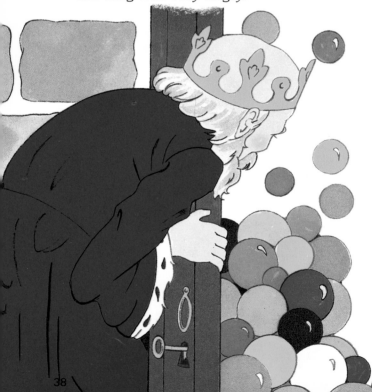

He called his magic bubble pipe men. Turning to the first one he said, "Blow me a green bubble."

The man tried, but no green bubble came. So the king turned to the next one, and the next one, all down the line.

Not one could blow a green bubble!

"Does no one know the secret of the green bubble?" he asked.

A servant spoke up. "It is whispered, Your Majesty," he said, "that the wizard has as his prisoners two butterflies who hold the secret. Whoever sets them free will then know what it is."

"Good," said the king. "Make ready, we will go tonight."

So that night they set off for the wizard's castle. The wizard must have heard of their coming, for he was waiting for them.

"Ha, ha," he chuckled, "so you have come for the secret. Well, you will not get it, for it is well guarded, and besides, you have no magic to help you, so be off with you."

Now the wizard was only a little man and the king tried to grab him. But the wizard was not to be caught so easily. He jumped up and down twice, crossed his arms and quickly turned into a lion.

The servant stood in front of the king to protect him and lifted his club to strike. But the wizard sprang right over their heads and then stood snarling at them.

The king realised that unless he did something soon the wizard would have them at his mercy.

Would he never learn the secret?

The wizard — who was now a lion of course — was getting ready to spring.

Suddenly the king had an idea and he turned to the wizard. "You say you are more powerful than I?" he said.

"That is true," snarled the wizard.

"Then," said the king, "turn yourself into a fish, as I could before I lost my magic powers."

"Easy," snarled the wizard, and without thinking, quickly turned into a fish.

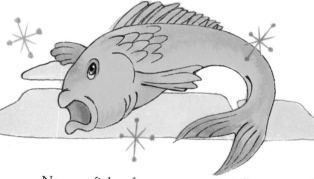

Now a fish of course cannot live out of water, and before the wizard realised his mistake he was lying gasping and helpless.

"Now for the secret," said the king to his servant, and they ran past the helpless wizard and into the castle.

They soon found the two butterfly prisoners.

The king set them free. One was a beautiful golden yellow and the other a beautiful blue.

"Now you are free," said the king, "tell us the secret of the green bubble."

But neither of them could speak!

Instead they stood close to one another and beat their wings together until they looked like one — and the colour they made was GREEN!

The king laughed so much his crown fell off. "So *that's* the secret," he said. "Yellow and blue makes green."

"Yellow and blue makes green," said the servant, copying the king.

The king looked at the two butterflies. "You will be well rewarded," he said, "and now, back to the palace, but before we go I must see that the wizard is all right."

And he did.

Then back to the palace they went, singing:

"Yellow and blue makes green,
Yellow and blue makes green,
All the time the secret's been
Yellow and blue makes green."

The king told his magic bubble pipe men the secret, and they made a big green bubble. The king then tried his magic, and it worked.

He was so pleased that he held a big party.

People came from miles around to hear the story and to see the green bubble, which lay on the table between the two butterflies, who were the guests of honour.

The wizard? He was never seen again.

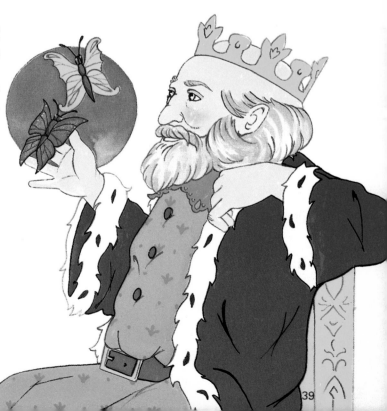

The Biscuit Tree

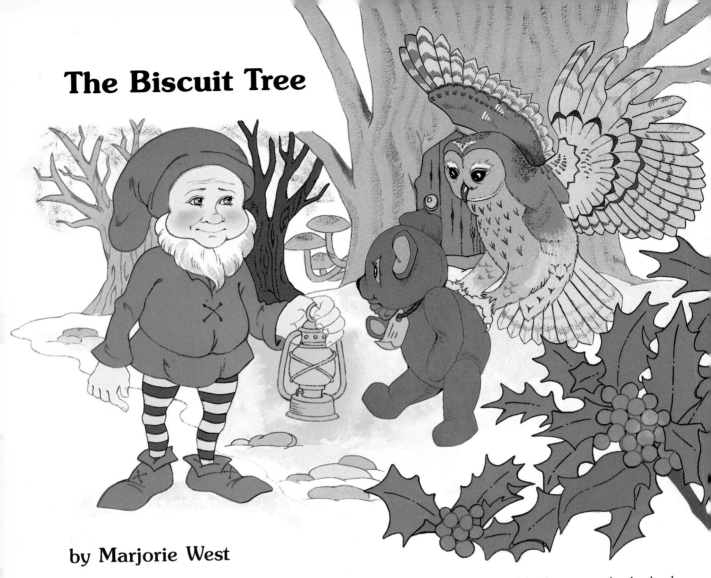

by Marjorie West

Red the dwarf opened the front door of Oak Tree Cottage. A gust of icy wind blew in, shaking the tip of his jelly bag hat, and Red shivered in his pointed little shoes.

"Help me!" someone was calling from the hollybushes.

Red looked longingly at his nice warm fire, took down his lantern, and trudged out into the snow. Holding the lantern high, he saw a small brown teddy bear hanging from the branches. The little toy was nearly frozen stiff. "I'm too short to reach you," Red said. "I'll have to fetch a ladder."

Just then Mr Owl screeched. "Mr Owl, please come quickly," Red called.

Mr Owl's great wings flapped above. "What's the matter?" he asked crossly. He was cold and hungry. Then he saw the frightened little teddy bear, and plucked him quickly off the bush and dropped him at Red's feet.

"Don't leave him there, bring him indoors," Red said. "We will all have some supper."

Back in Oak Tree Cottage they were sitting round the fire, sipping hot tomato soup, when Mr Owl bent forward and took hold of a soggy piece of cardboard tied round the little bear's neck.

"A woolly bear, for Brenda. With love from Santa Claus," he read. "Well, well, so you have fallen off Santa's sleigh."

Woolly Bear nodded sadly. "Then it must be Christmas Eve," said Red. "Let's have a party."

"Parties must wait," Mr Owl said wisely.

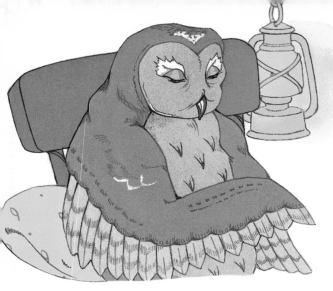

"We have come to ask a favour," Mr Owl said. "Woolly Bear has fallen from Santa Claus's sleigh. This label says he is for Brenda, but we don't know where she lives."

"Mother Cat will help you," the woodcutter said. "Take them to the Biscuit Tree, Mother Cat."

They followed Mother Cat into the garden, and she led them to the Biscuit Tree. Among its branches grew biscuits of all shapes, sizes and colours.

"Our duty is to Santa Claus. We must find Brenda, before daybreak. But how?"

Mr Owl relaxed in his chair and closed his eyes. All was quiet for a while, except for the wind in the chimney and the hissing from the lamp. Woolly Bear soon fell fast asleep.

Some time later, Mr Owl sat up, blinking. "I have it," he said, getting up from his chair. "We must go to the woodcutter's." At that, he flew off, screeching at the others to follow.

The woodcutter was very pleased to have visitors on Christmas Eve. "Come in and warm yourselves," he said, moving three beautiful black and white cats off the hearth where they had been snoozing.

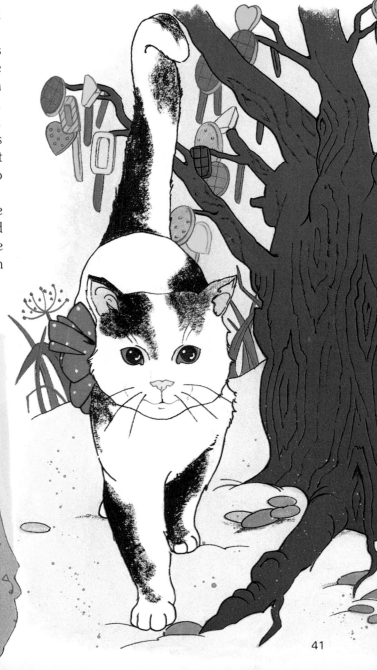

Woolly Bear's eyes were glued to a pretty little white biscuit. It was decorated with silver balls, and was dangling in front of his nose. He did not hear Mother Cat say, "You must look for one very special biscuit, with 'EAT ME' written on it."

The others were so busy searching for the biscuit that they didn't see Woolly Bear picking the pretty biscuit and eating it. Until Red let out a yell. He had turned to see a very hazy Woolly Bear, a half-eaten biscuit in his paw. The haze cleared, and Woolly Bear had gone!

Mother Cat was solemn. "If he has eaten one of the forbidden biscuits, we may never hear of Woolly Bear again. The tree goblins will have taken him. They will keep him prisoner, and make him do all their work."

They hunted high and low among the tree's branches, but the 'EAT ME' biscuit was nowhere to be seen. "There goes our last chance of finding Woolly Bear," said Mother Cat. "Without the biscuit, we have no magic powers to rescue him."

Dawn was breaking. "What's that noise?" Mr Owl asked, listening.

"Sleigh bells," said Red sadly. "We are too late. That's Santa Claus on his way home."

Mr Owl flew off and landed on the moving sleigh beside Santa Claus. "It's about Woolly Bear," he said. "He has eaten a magic biscuit, and vanished."

Santa Claus smiled sleepily. He had had a very busy night. "You must be mistaken. Why, only a few minutes ago, I put Woolly Bear down a chimney."

The clever, naughty little bear had seen and eaten the 'EAT ME' biscuit, and made his wish to be back on Santa's sleigh. Santa had not even missed him.

"No wonder we couldn't find the magic biscuit!" said Red, on their way home. "Mr Owl, it's Christmas Day, let's have a party." And this time Mr Owl agreed.

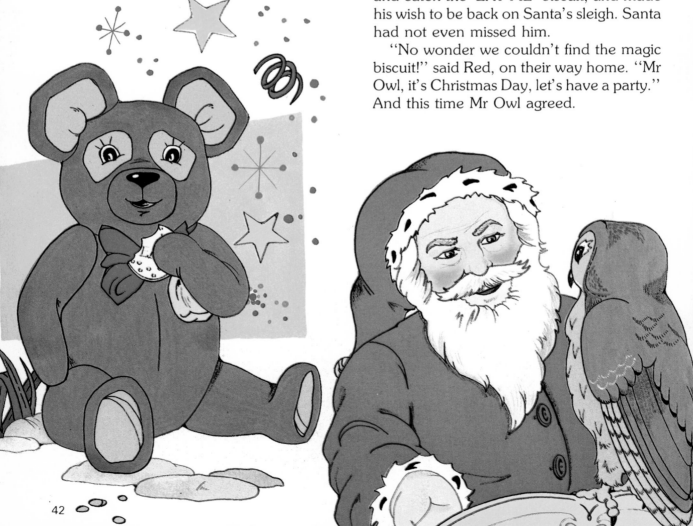

The Mouse Family Move House

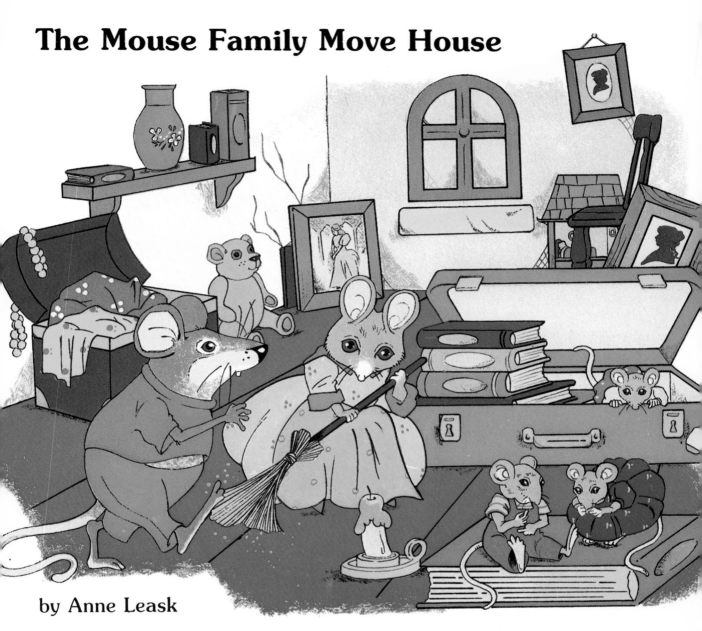

by Anne Leask

Meeny, Miny and Mo were three baby brown mice who lived with their mother and father in Professor Paperchase's dark, dusty attic.

Their house was a half-open suitcase full of old books. Father Mouse, with his strong teeth, had gnawed a little doorway in the suitcase so that Meeny, Miny and Mo could get in and out easily when they wanted to play in the attic.

Meeny, Miny and Mo were quite happy, but Mother Mouse often worried about them.

"It's so bad for their health to be cooped up in a stuffy attic all the time!" she complained to Father Mouse. "And it can't be good for their digestion to eat so much dry paper. They'll grow up into bookworms instead of mice, by the time they've nibbled through all these books! How I wish we could move to the country where they would get some fresh air, and more nourishing food to eat!"

Father Mouse agreed. But Meeny, Miny and Mo were too small to set out on a long journey to the country. "Perhaps when

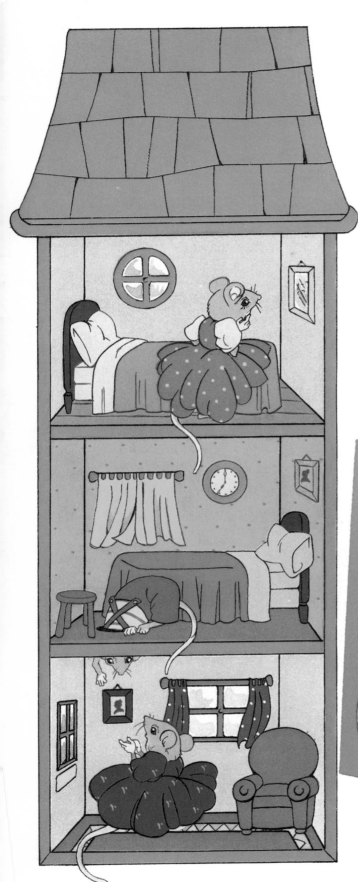

they're older," he said, "we might be able to move out of the town."

One day there was a great commotion in Professor Paperchase's home. Furniture bumped across the floor, and heavy footsteps tramped through the house.

Then the footsteps came nearer. Somebody was climbing the attic stairs.

Meeny, Miny and Mo were playing inside a doll's house, which had belonged to Professor Paperchase's children when they were small. "Quick!" called Mother Mouse. "Into the suitcase!"

They were not a moment too soon. With a thud, the lid slammed shut, just missing Mo's tail. The suitcase was carried downstairs, with the frightened mouse family slithering about inside, and put into a big van.

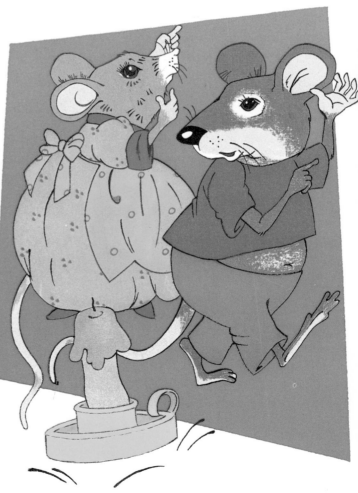

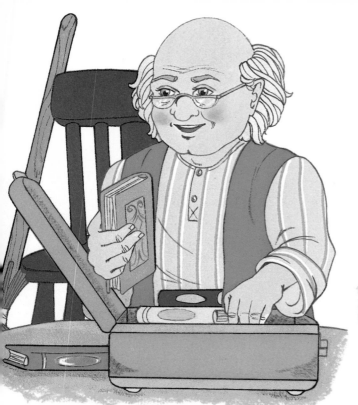

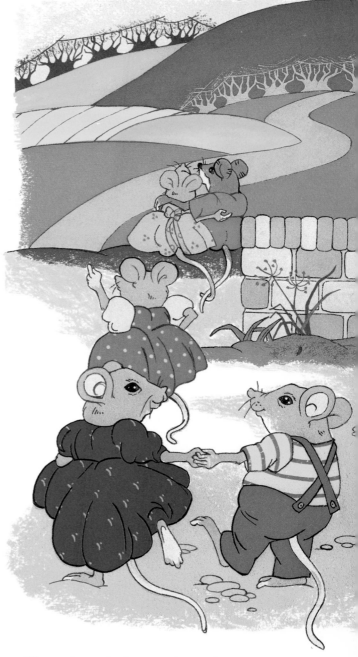

For hours, it seemed, they were shaken and jolted till they ached all over. They clung together, wondering what was going to happen to them until, at last, the van stopped.

The suitcase was taken out and flung down on a hard floor – then all was quiet.

The bruised mice felt themselves carefully to make sure that no bones were broken. Then Father Mouse decided to go and explore. "Do be careful!" begged Mother Mouse anxiously. "I'm sure I can smell cat!"

Just as Meeny, Miny and Mo were getting tired of being shut inside the suitcase, Father Mouse returned, beaming from whisker to whisker.

"Your wish has come true!" he told Mother Mouse. "We have moved to the country – with Professor Paperchase, and all his furniture!"

His family squeaked with excitement. And before Professor Paperchase could unpack the suitcase, the Mouse family had slipped out through an open door, to look for a new house.

They found the perfect place – in a woodshed in the garden. Under the door was a space, big enough to let a mouse squeeze through, but safe from prowling cats. Inside, there were woodshavings to build a snug nest, and over the garden wall lay a field of ripe corn. Mother Mouse's mouth watered just to look at it.

"No more dusty books for dinner," she said happily. "We're going to be country mice for a change!"

The Frog Who Couldn't Hop

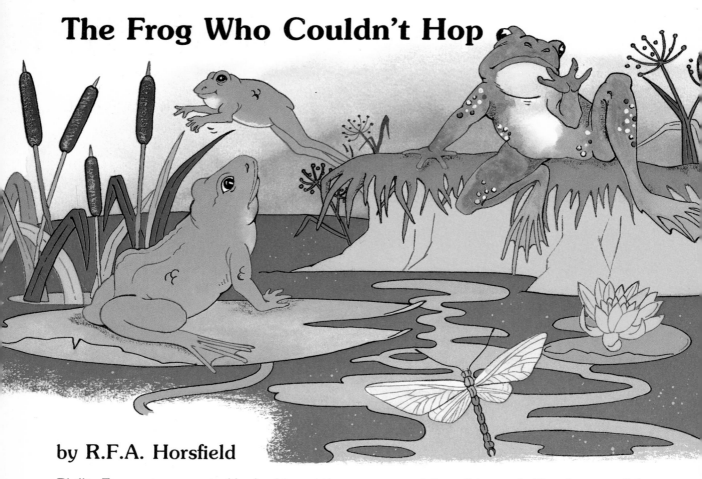

by R.F.A. Horsfield

Phillip Frog sat on a waterlily, looking at the water. It was a hot summer's day and the river looked cool and inviting. Just right for a swim. But Phillip didn't feel like swimming. "All I do is swim," he complained aloud. "And what I *really* want to do is hop."

"Well, hop over here then, and have a chat," said a voice from the river bank. Phillip looked up and saw Tommy Toad who had made his way down to the water's edge for a drink.

"I can't," he said sadly. "That's just it. I can't hop."

"Can't hop?" asked Tommy in surprise. "Why, I thought *all* frogs could hop."

"Well, *I* can't," replied Phillip. "All I can do is crawl. Or swim. And I'm fed up with crawling and swimming. I want to be like other frogs and hop around for a change."

Tommy took a sip of water and stretched his legs. "Nothing wrong with crawling, young fellow," he said. "Look at me. I do it all the time, don't I? Takes a bit longer, perhaps, but I get there just the same."

"But I'm not a toad," protested Phillip. "I suppose if I was, I'd just crawl under a stone and sleep all day like you seem to do. I'm a frog, and frogs are supposed to hop, aren't they? All my brothers and sisters can hop. They've been hopping ever since they stopped being tadpoles. Everyone hops, except me. I just sit here on this dull old waterlily and look at the river. I can swim all right, but I'm fed up with swimming. I want to hop!"

Tommy shook his head sadly and crawled under a dockleaf. Phillip sat on his waterlily and looked around him. His brothers and sisters, aunts and uncles, grandmothers and grandfathers were all hopping about like mad, having a fine old time. His younger sister, Freda, stopped hopping and called to him. "Come over and play with us, Phillip," she cried. "It's lovely here, in the mud."

But Phillip didn't answer. He felt sad and lonely. None of the other frogs wanted to come and sit on the waterlily and talk to him. That was far too dull for them. All they wanted to do was hop. And hop. And hop. A little tear formed in his eye and trickled down his face.

Tommy Toad wished that he could help Phillip, but he had no idea of how to teach a frog to hop. He was just dozing off when he heard Phillip cry out.

"Tommy! Tommy! The waterlily is moving!"

Tommy Toad looked up quickly. The lily was indeed moving. It was jiggling and joggling in a way that waterlilies do not usually move. And Phillip was crouched in the middle of one of the big leaves, his eyes wide with fright. Tommy began to crawl to the water's edge.

"Oh, do hurry up," cried Phillip. "Something terrible is happening, I'm sure!"

"I *am* hurrying," replied Tommy, a little crossly. "I'm doing my best."

All the other frogs had seen the lily moving, too. "Jump in and swim, Phillip!" cried Freda. "It's not far to the bank."

But Phillip wouldn't move an inch. He just sat there, right in the middle of the waterlily, holding on for dear life. And then, to his horror, a shape began to rise from the water. At first there was just a large, green hump. Then a fin. And, finally, the long, wicked face of Percy Pike, his beady eyes fixed on Phillip, and his wide, fierce mouth open just enough to show his sharp white teeth.

"Gnarrrrrrrr!" cried Percy Pike.

"Help!" yelled Phillip in a shrill voice. And then he hopped! And, because he was facing Percy Pike, he didn't hop forward. He hopped backwards! A terrific hop which sent him flying high over the heads of all the other frogs who just sat and watched in wonder as he landed with a loud plop in the mud.

"Why, Phillip!" cried Freda. "You did it! You actually hopped! And backwards too! I don't believe there's another frog in the world who can hop backwards!"

"Nothing to it, really," said Phillip modestly. "Nothing at all." But he smiled, just the same. It was nice to be famous. And, from that day on, he never stopped hopping. Backwards, of course!

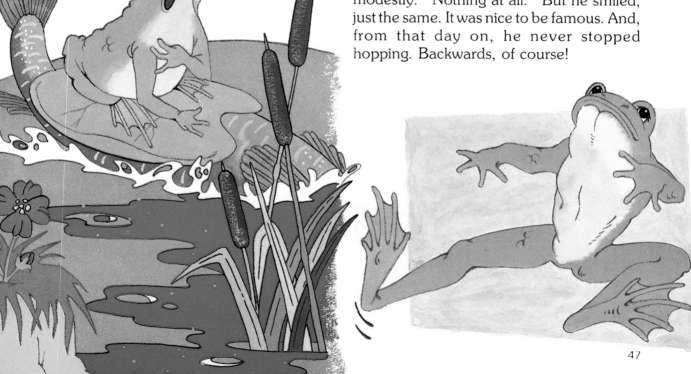

Timbaree

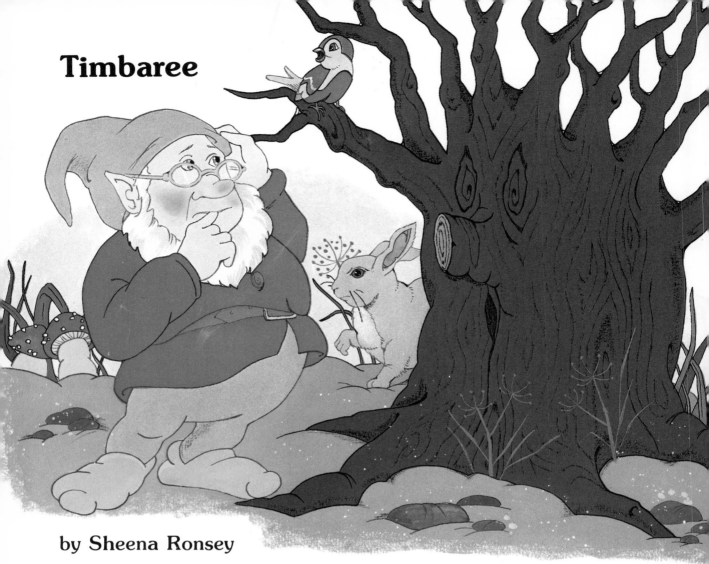

by Sheena Ronsey

Jindle the gnome whistled cheerfully. He was looking forward to seeing his friends the wood pixies again, and he listened for their voices among the trees. Then he noticed something very strange. When he stopped whistling, there was nothing to be heard but his own footsteps, and when he stood still there was no sound at all. The forest was too quiet. Whatever could be wrong?

"Why aren't you singing?" he asked some birds.

"Timbaree," they twittered, and hopped away.

"Why aren't you whispering?" he asked the trees.

"Timbaree," they sighed.

What has happened to Timbaree? wondered the gnome. It must be something terrible to make the birds and trees so unhappy. He hurried towards the pixie village.

"Hello, Jindle," said a pixie. "I'm sorry there will be no singing or dancing tonight, but you are welcome to stay with us as usual."

"What is the matter?" asked Jindle.

"Timbaree has been stolen away," said the pixie. "Goblins came down from the Blue Mountain and caught her in their net." Tears began to trickle down his face. "Not even the nightingales could sing as sweetly as Timbaree."

That news made Jindle feel like crying too. He wished he could help, but he was only a poor, old gnome, so what could he do? He went to the pixies' meeting, but he

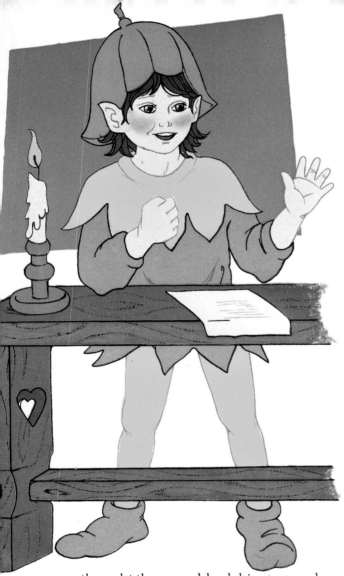

the pixies, and poor Jindle was pushed to the front.

He was a very worried gnome at that moment. All gnomes like to look wise, and some of them really are wise, but Jindle did not count himself among the wise ones. It was terrible to feel all those eyes watching him, and to know that everyone was waiting for him to speak.

"Well," said Jindle. "First I need to know the facts." He hoped that sounded grand enough. "How many goblins are there?"

"Lots!" called some pixies.

"Dozens!" cried others.

"Three," said the Chief Pixie firmly.

"Only three!" said Jindle.

"They're bigger than we are," said the pixies. "We're only as high as their knees." They thought Jindle was wondering why so many pixies were afraid of only three goblins, and they did not like it.

The gnome's face went red. He had not meant to be rude. If only he could think of something clever to say.

"Why did they do it?" he asked.

"Why?" said the pixies. "Why steal her? We don't know."

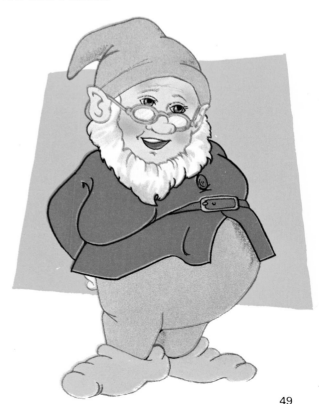

never thought they would ask him to speak.

"We are here to plan the rescue of Timbaree," said the Chief Pixie.

"Yes, yes," shouted all the pixies.

The Chief Pixie had to bang on the table for quiet. "Some of you followed the goblins to the Blue Mountain," he said.

"Yes." A pixie stood up. "When we went near the gate the goblins chased us with sticks and nets. We don't know what they have done with Timbaree."

Everybody started talking, and the Chief Pixie banged the table again. Then he asked if anyone had ideas about what to do next.

"Jindle the gnome is here," called one pixie. "Gnomes are always wise. He'll tell us what to do."

"Yes, yes. Hurrah for Jindle," shouted

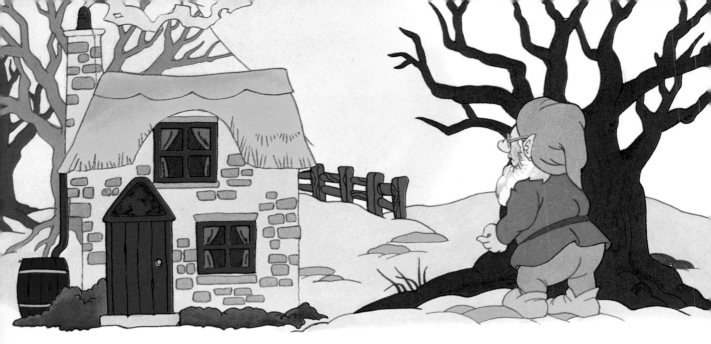

"Perhaps they want a servant," said one.

"Do goblins eat pixies?" asked another.

"No!" Jindle *did* know that. "Sometimes they let their prisoners go if people give them gold," he said.

"We'll send a messenger to ask them," said the Chief Pixie. "Who will go?"

The pixies suddenly became very quiet. Go and speak to the goblins? Not me, each of them thought, somebody else can do it.

"I will go," said Jindle.

The pixies cheered him loudly. They kept him company as far as the edge of the forest, then the gnome went on alone to the goblins' house. He knocked at the door, and nearly fainted with fright when it opened. He had never seen any creatures as ugly as those goblins. They were hideous. He wanted to run away, but he remembered Timbaree.

"It's a gnome," said the goblins. "Come in."

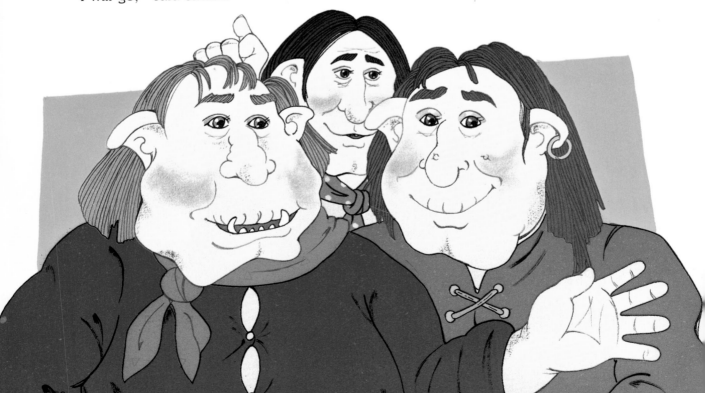

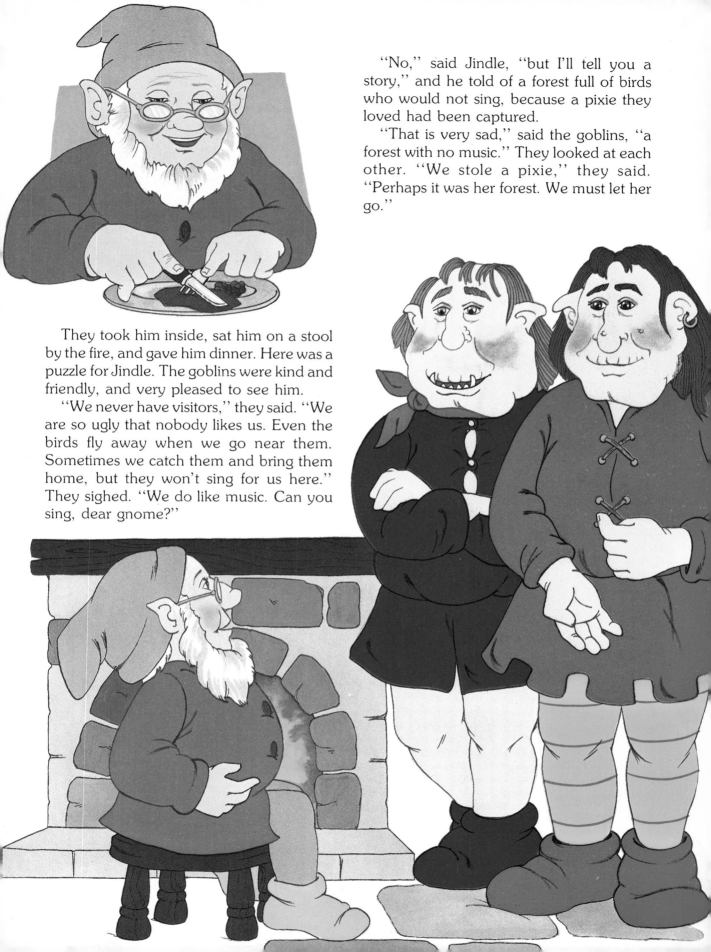

"No," said Jindle, "but I'll tell you a story," and he told of a forest full of birds who would not sing, because a pixie they loved had been captured.

"That is very sad," said the goblins, "a forest with no music." They looked at each other. "We stole a pixie," they said. "Perhaps it was her forest. We must let her go."

They took him inside, sat him on a stool by the fire, and gave him dinner. Here was a puzzle for Jindle. The goblins were kind and friendly, and very pleased to see him.

"We never have visitors," they said. "We are so ugly that nobody likes us. Even the birds fly away when we go near them. Sometimes we catch them and bring them home, but they won't sing for us here." They sighed. "We do like music. Can you sing, dear gnome?"

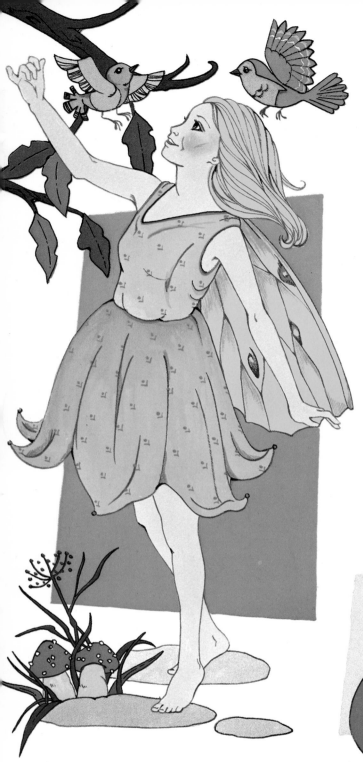

At the edge of the forest Timbaree started to sing for joy. The birds heard her and joined in, spreading the news. The pixies sang and danced in the village streets while the goblins stood and listened. It was the most wonderful music they had ever heard. Somebody coughed, and the goblins looked down.

"Here is the Chief Pixie," said Jindle.

"Would you goblins like to build a house near our village?" said the Chief Pixie nervously. He did not much like this plan of Jindle's.

The goblins were thrilled. Now they could hear music every day.

"No more catching birds," warned Jindle. "Or pixies."

"Oh no," said the goblins. "We always wanted to be friends, but nobody listened until you came."

"Gnomes are wise people," said the Chief Pixie.

Jindle laughed. Perhaps he *was* wise, after all!

One of the goblins fetched Timbaree. They begged her to sing for them before she went home. "If only we could hear such lovely music every day," said the goblins.

"Come back with us," said Jindle. "The birds will surely sing to welcome Timbaree. But leave your nets behind."

The Jumbo Jumble

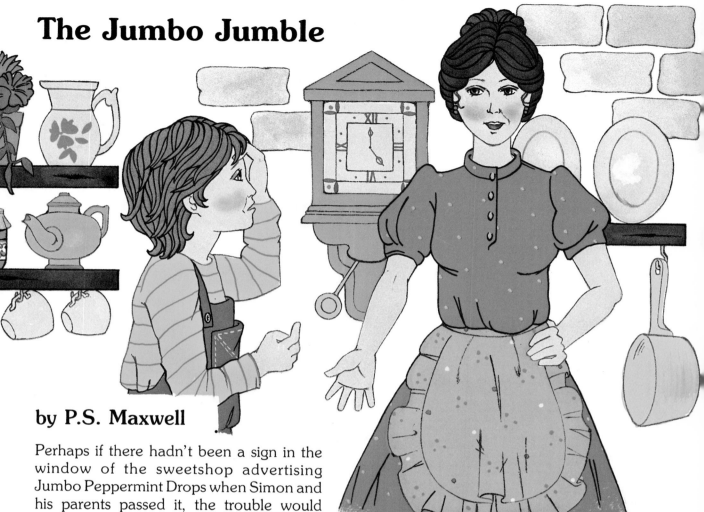

by P.S. Maxwell

Perhaps if there hadn't been a sign in the window of the sweetshop advertising Jumbo Peppermint Drops when Simon and his parents passed it, the trouble would never have happened. Simon loved peppermints, so when he saw the sign he had to go in and buy some.

"Look how they've spelt it on the packet," he said as he came out of the shop with his sweets.

"Jumble Peppermint Drops," read his mother.

"Just a misprint, I expect," said his father. "They'll taste just as good."

But he didn't have one when Simon offered him one, and nor did Simon's mother. This was probably just as well, or things might have been three times as bad. Simon ate all the Jumble Peppermint Drops himself.

It wasn't till Simon had eaten all of them that it was clear that something was rather wrong.

"What would you like for tea, Simon?" asked his mother when they got back home again.

"Jamberly jomberly," replied Simon.

"Pardon?" asked his mother.

"Jamberly jomberly," Simon repeated.

"I don't think I've heard of that, dear," his mother said carefully. "What's it made of?"

"Jig-a-jiggle joggy jag," said Simon.

"Simon dear, I think you're being a bit silly," said his mother. "I can't give you what you want for tea if you won't tell me what it is."

"Woggledy dongle," said Simon unhappily.

"Well, you can just have sausages and like it," said his mother impatiently.

"What's the trouble?" asked his father, coming into the kitchen at that moment. "What's wrong with sausages for tea?"

"It's Simon being silly," explained his mother.

"Argle bargle blump!" said Simon indignantly.

"I see what you mean," agreed his father.

"Binky lobble," said Simon, almost in tears.

"Hold on a minute," said his father. "I think something really is wrong."

"Jumbley mumbley reebledum," said Simon.

"I know what it is," said his father. "He's eaten those Jumble Peppermint Drops and they've jumbled up his speech."

"Fratchity millwackit," agreed Simon, nodding furiously.

It was very worrying. Simon found it almost impossible to make himself understood. All he could do was point, or nod, or shake his head.

"Perhaps it will wear off in time," said his father, but it didn't.

"It's no good, Simon," said his mother at last. "Aunty Margaret is coming to stay tomorrow, and we don't want her to hear you talking like this."

"Surbuddy noople," agreed Simon.

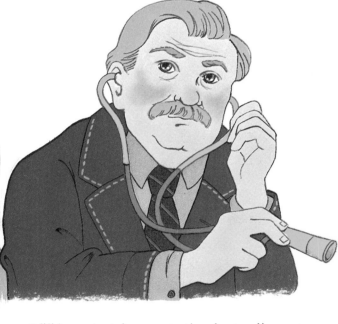

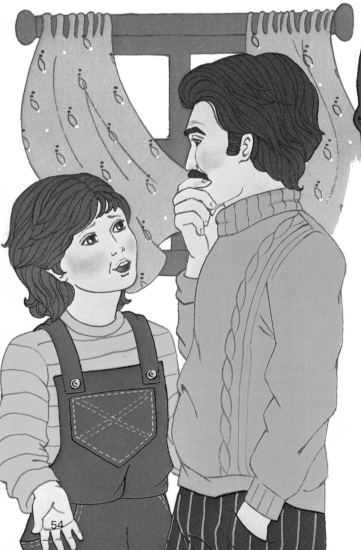

"I'll have to take you to the doctor," went on his mother, "and see if he can sort out your difficulty."

An hour later, they were in the doctor's surgery.

"Now, Simon, what's the problem?" asked the doctor brightly.

"He's having difficulty with his speech," said Simon's mother quickly before Simon had a chance to reply.

"Perhaps we would do better if Simon told me himself," suggested the doctor.

"Yankle macfilliman oppertop mooble," said Simon. "Yeedle yerdle," he added helpfully.

"Dear me," said the doctor. "How long has he been like this, Mrs Torrington?" The doctor had decided that after all it would be easier if Simon's mother told him.

"Ever since he ate a packet of Jumble Peppermint Drops last week," replied his mother.

"Dear me," said the doctor again, and began peering down Simon's throat. "Say ah."

"Oog," said Simon.

"Is he going to be all right, Doctor?" asked Simon's mother.

"Yes . . . I think so," replied the doctor, but he didn't sound very sure.

"Mingwibble yumple gramp," said Simon.

"Quite so," said the doctor. "I'm sure this is very difficult for you, Mrs Torrington."

"It is," said Simon's mother.

"Zoggermoof," added Simon, just so the doctor would understand.

"Well, well," said the doctor, getting up nervously, "I think the best thing you can do is come back and see me next week if there's no change."

Simon's mother was about to say something, but the doctor opened the door and said, "Good bye," very loudly and firmly. Simon and his mother returned home.

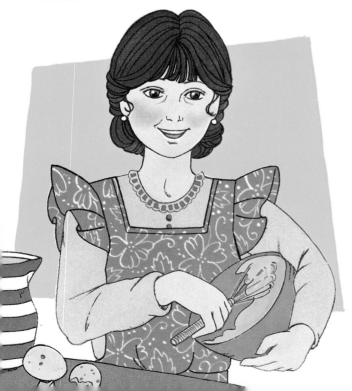

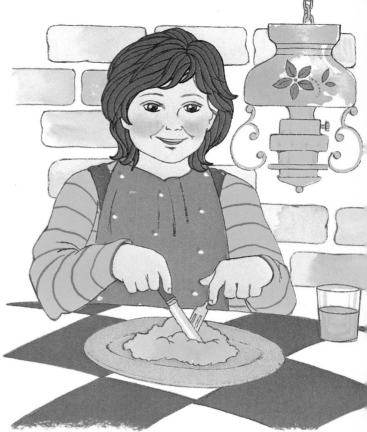

Next day, Simon's Aunty Margaret arrived.

"Try not to say anthing unless you have to," his mother told him.

"Oable tooblip," promised Simon.

Of course, that was easier said than done. Aunty Margaret kept asking Simon lots of questions, and really wanted *him* to answer, not his mother. Finally, she did hear Simon talk, and was told the whole story of the Jumble Peppermint Drops. She didn't seem the least bit concerned.

"Nothing to worry about," she said. "Scrambled egg. That'll cure him."

"Scrambled egg?" asked Simon's mother.

"Rumble tumble?" asked Simon.

"Yes," replied Aunty Margaret. "The peppermints jumbled up his speech and the scrambled egg will unscramble it."

One plate of scrambled egg later, Simon was talking quite normally again.

"That's better," he sighed with relief. "I think it will be a long time before I eat peppermints again."

Silas, the Snake, Does a Good Turn

by Anne Leask

Silas was a slippery, slithery brown snake who lived in the jungle, in a banana tree with big, feathery leaves. He would coil himself round the tree till he looked just like a twisted brown branch. Then he would unwind his coils and hang down like a long, brown rope, to watch the monkey children playing football with a hairy coconut.

His bright, beady eyes glittered with excitement, and his forked tongue flicked in and out of his mouth. He longed to join in their games, but whenever he came too near, Mother Monkey said to her children, "Run along now, no more football! Silas is here and snakes can bite, you know!"

It was the same when he slithered through the tall bamboo canes to where the tiger cubs played hide-and-seek. When their mother saw Silas, she growled, "Look

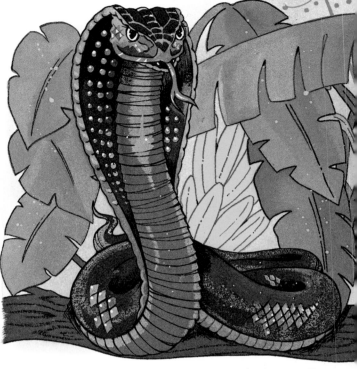

out! Here comes Silas!" and they all scampered away.

Even when Silas slid up the trunk of a tree, the parrots scolded, chattering a warning to each other, and flew off to another tree.

Poor Silas just couldn't understand it at all. He didn't want to bite anyone! All he wanted was someone to play with, for he often felt very lonely.

One hot day, all the animals in the jungle were having an afternoon nap. The monkeys were sound asleep under a coconut palm, Silas was curled up in a fork of the banana tree, dozing peacefully, and there wasn't a sound to be heard.

Suddenly, Silas was wakened by a soft, whimpering noise nearby. Had he been dreaming? No, there it was again, high up in the banana tree.

He lifted his smooth, flat head, and stared with his beady eyes. There, at the top of the tree, clinging to a very thin branch, which

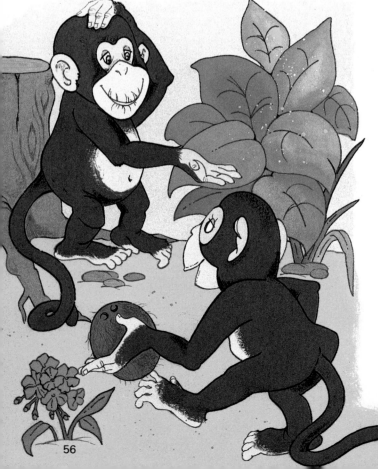

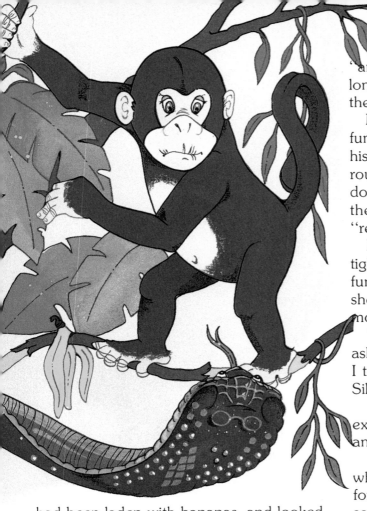

"and hang down as far as I can stretch, like a long rope. Then you can slide down right to the ground."

Mathilda cheered up. That sounded great fun! She watched eagerly while Silas flicked his tail up beside her, knotting it tightly round the branch. Then the rest of him slid down the tree, till his head was almost on the ground. "Now then," he told her, "ready, steady, go!"

Mathilda gripped his slithery, scaly body tightly with her little pink hands. "Ooh, what fun this is!" she cried, and with a *whoosh*! she was at the bottom of the tree, just as her mother woke from her nap.

"Where have you been, Mathilda?" asked her mother crossly. "How often have I told you never to go away by yourself? Silas might find you!"

"But, Mother," said Mathilda, "that's exactly what happened. Silas *did* find me, and brought me safely back!"

Silas was busy untying the knot in his tail when Mother Monkey came to thank him for helping Mathilda. "I'm sorry we've been so unkind to you, Silas," she apologised, "but please come and drink some coconut milk with us, and we'll be friends."

After that, Silas was often to be seen giving swings to the monkey children, and tying knots in his tail to amuse them. And he was never lonely again.

had been laden with bananas, and looked as if it were going to break any moment, was Mathilda, the youngest of Mother Monkey's children. She was all alone, shivering with fright as she looked at the ground, which seemed to be an awfully long way down.

"What are you doing up there, Mathilda?" asked Silas curiously. "You're much too small to be at the top of a big tree all by yourself!"

Mathilda looked ashamed. "Well, you see," she explained, "I felt hungry, and the bananas on this tree are so delicious that I thought I would have a little snack while everybody else was asleep." She rubbed her tummy. "Oh, dear, I wish I hadn't eaten so many bananas! I really don't feel very well. And I don't know how I'm going to get down from this branch!"

Silas scratched his head with the tip of his tail, and thought hard for a minute or two. Then he had an idea. "I'll twist my tail round the branch where you're sitting," he said,

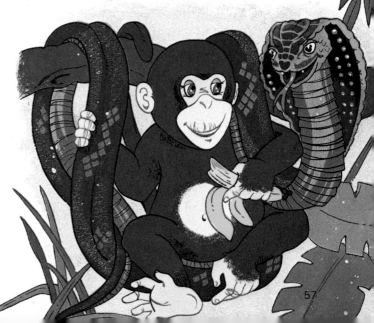

57

Marvin the Supermouse

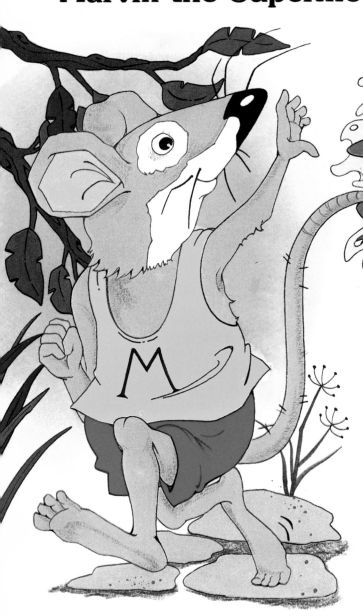

by Derek Friedlander

"I'm Marvin, the strongest mouse in all the world!" shouted Marvin Mouse, and with a jump and a shout of CHEESERO he ran twice round his nest, rolled over backwards, then collapsed in a furry heap on the floor. This was Marvin Woodmouse, the strongest mouse in all of Fol-Hollow; perhaps in all the world.

Now all the creatures liked Marvin. He was so small that he never caused any real trouble. He would wake up every morning, pull on his blue shorts, and begin his daily exercises: Pressups, Mouseups, Tail Wagging, Running on the Tabletop and, if Marvin was feeling extra strong, Cracking the Walnut with Bare Hands!

Marvin was running around the wood one morning. "Wake up, you lazy things, keep fit, keep fit!" shouted Marvin as he sped past the frogs. "Good morning, frogs, lovely day for a jog!"

"Yes, but we would rather be frogs than jog," giggled the frogs, but Marvin had already disappeared.

"Wake up, you lazy things!" shouted Marvin again, jumping up and down on top of the rabbit warren.

After a few minutes of jogging on the spot a carrot came flying out of the warren and a voice boomed out, "That's the only exercise you'll get from us!" The carrot hit Marvin square on the nose and he fell down. When he got up again and brushed the dust from his furry nose, he was greeted by a group of angry rabbits. "Look, it's that silly mouse, and he's wearing blue shorts," said the rabbits, and they all began to laugh.

This made the woodmouse very angry, and before he could control his temper, he issued a challenge: "I'm so strong I could pull you all over!"

The rabbits closed around Marvin and before he could say SMELLY CHEESE *they* issued a challenge; they challenged Marvin to a tug of war, not with a rabbit, but with an oak tree!

When Marvin got home the thought of what he had to do was just too much for him and, as all mice do when they are in trouble, Marvin curled up into a furry ball and fell fast asleep.

The next day Marvin woke early. It was still dark outside, but he was determined to win the tug of war with the oak tree, so he

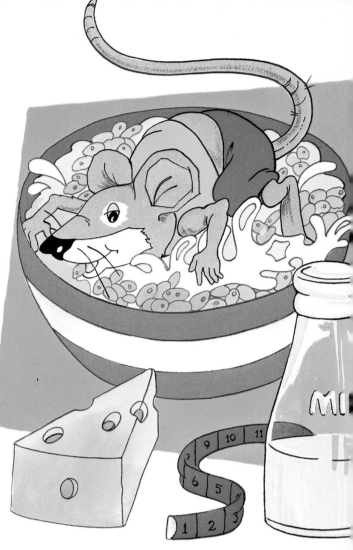

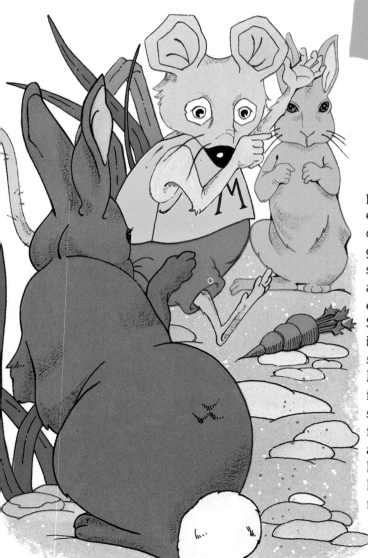

pulled on his blue shorts and began his exercises. After training was over he decided that he would have to eat lots of good healthy food to make himself extra strong. He put oats and mouse crispies into a bowl, then poured some fresh mouse-milk on top, and before you could say SUPERMOUSE, Marvin dived head first into his bowl of food! Round and round swam the mouse and as he did so he went MUNCH, MUNCH, MUNCH. Finally all his food was gone, and Marvin even ate a special piece of cheese that he was saving for Christmas. He took his tape measure and measured all his muscles. He measured his arms, his legs, his feet, but although he had eaten all that food he had not grown, not even an inch!

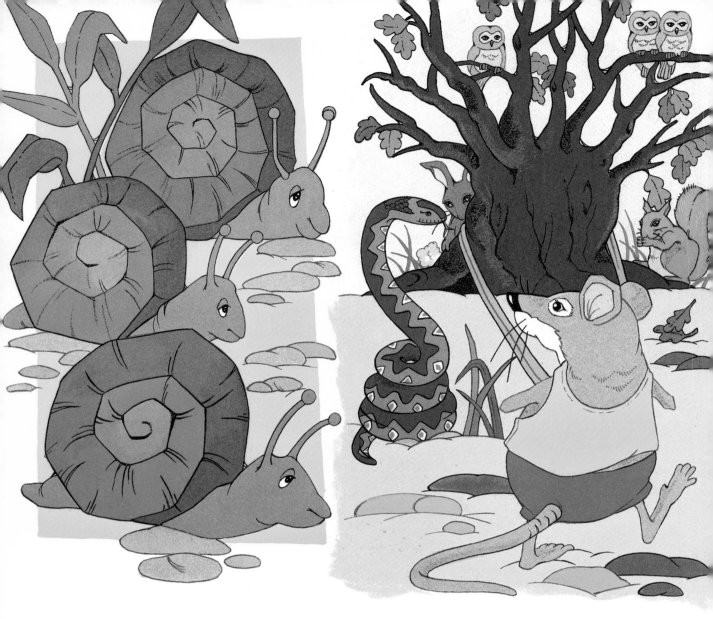

Marvin stuck his hands in his ears and began to think, in fact he thought so hard that he fell off his chair and rolled across the floor and stopped against his wooden chest. It was then that he had an amazing idea. Marvin opened his chest and inside he found an old pair of braces. He spent the rest of the day making them into a very special rope.

On the day of the contest everybody travelled to Fol-Hollow to watch. The snails had set out a day earlier than everybody else because they moved so slowly; some even hitched a lift on a badger's back. All around the tree stood rabbits, squirrels, stoats, hedgehogs and foxes (who had been given the job of organising the crowd). The snakes were going to be the judges, because they said they could measure, as they were the longest.

The last to arrive was Marvin. Everyone cheered when they saw him. He walked up to the tree, bowed to it, then tied his special rope around the trunk. Sitting in the tree were three owls, but Marvin said that they could stay, as they would probably help him keep his balance. Everybody cheered again, and the chief snake began to speak. "If Marvin crosses this line he will have pulled the tree more than five inches,

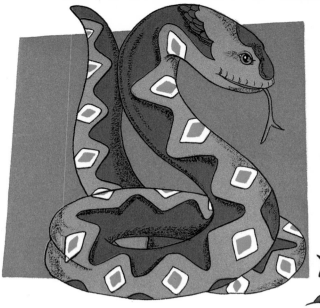

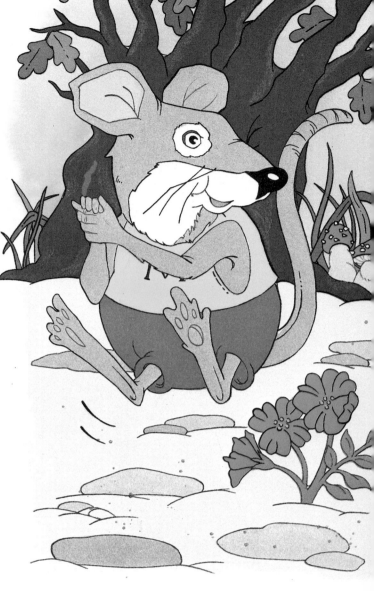

making Marvin the strongest mouse in all of Fol-Hollow — and in all the world!'' Everybody cheered again and Marvin got ready to pull.

The crowd fell silent and even the wind hushed a little, then the chief snake shouted, "Ready, steady, pull!" and Marvin dug in his little mouse heels and began to heave.

Nothing happened and it looked as though the oak tree would win. The crowd shouted, "Heave!" but still Marvin did not move.

"If only they knew what my rope was made of," said Marvin to himself, and he pretended to strain and pull again. It was looking bad for the little woodmouse and the rabbits all started to laugh, when

suddenly Marvin let out a mighty shout of CHEESERO! and began to move backwards. Inch by inch he moved, pulling on the braces, until he crossed the line.

Everybody shouted and cheered, "Look, look, he's crossing the line, look!" Even the rabbits cheered and they rushed forward and grabbed Marvin and carried him off around Fol-Hollow, singing and cheering.

Meanwhile, sitting in the tree were the three owls, who knew that the tree had not moved even a mouse inch, but they were not going to say anthing to anybody. After all, it isn't every day that you see the strongest mouse in all the world, is it?

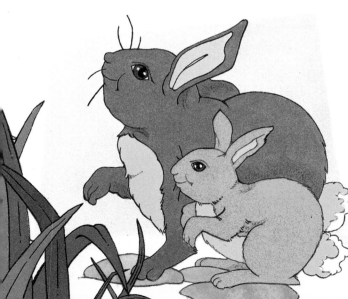

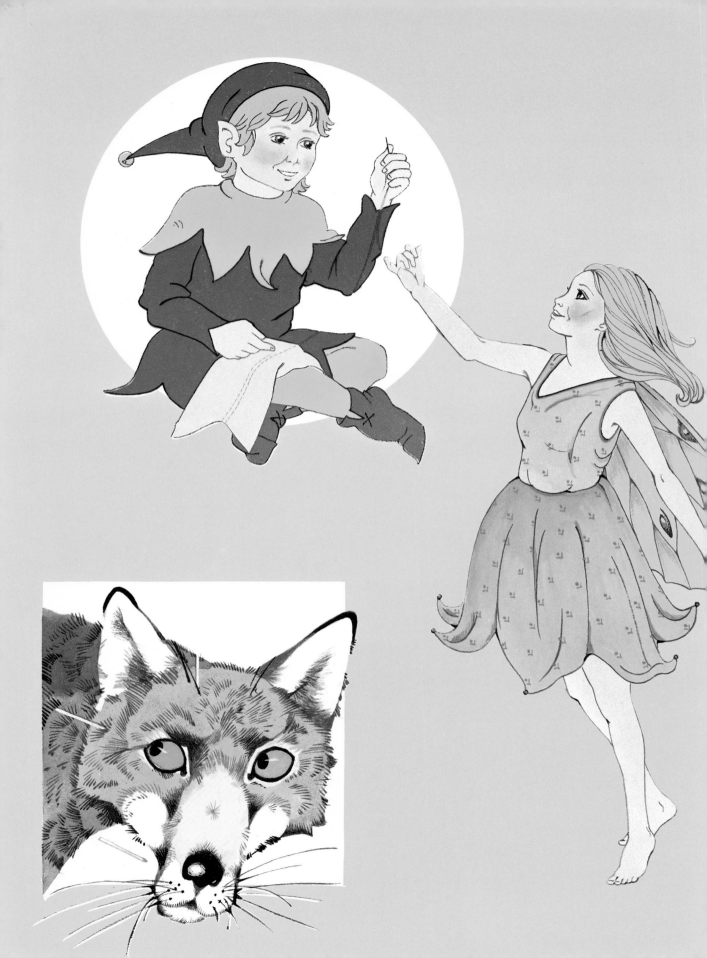